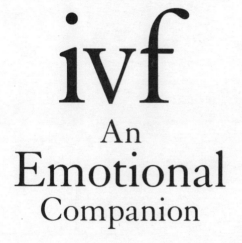

ivf

An
Emotional
Companion

ivf
An
Emotional
Companion

BRIGID MOSS

Collins

First published in 2011 by Collins
an imprint of HarperCollins*Publishers*
77–85 Fulham Palace Road
London W6 8JB

www.harpercollins.co.uk

1 3 5 7 9 10 8 6 4 2

Text © Brigid Moss 2011

The author asserts her moral right to
be identified as the author of this work

A catalogue record of this book is
available from the British Library

ISBN 978-0-00-741433-8

Printed and bound in Great Britain by
Clays Ltd, St Ives plc

MIX
Paper from
responsible sources
FSC® C007454

FSC™ is a non-profit international organisation established to promote
the responsible management of the world's forests. Products carrying the
FSC label are independently certified to assure consumers that they come
from forests that are managed to meet the social, economic and
ecological needs of present and future generations,
and other controlled sources.

Find out more about HarperCollins and the environment at
www.harpercollins.co.uk/green

Contents

· · · · · · · · · · · ·

Surviving IVF

Introduction

· · · · · · · · · · · ·

I don't know how long you've been trying for a baby, which fertility investigations or treatments you've had or what your chances are now of getting pregnant. You could just be thinking about having IVF, you might be a veteran IVF-er who's had multiple cycles, or you may be about to start out on your first cycle. Wherever you are on your IVF journey, this book is for you.

If I think back, I can still remember the feelings of inadequacy, shame and loneliness that I had when I couldn't get pregnant. That was my motivation for writing this book, a collection of stories from 22 amazing women who are sharing them because, like me, they remember how it feels to be among the one in six couples who experience infertility. Each one of them volunteered to tell her story because she wanted to let you and others know that IVF can be hard, but that you can get through it.

When I was first told I'd need IVF, almost six years ago, aged 35, I couldn't talk to anyone about my fertility problems.

Writing this book – admitting my infertility to everyone – and speaking to the women whose stories are told in these pages has been liberating for me. As one woman said to me, 'IVF and infertility need to be brought out into the open. Nobody should be ashamed any more.'

But back then, I didn't want anyone to feel sorry for me or pity me or gossip about me. I didn't want friends to think they couldn't tell me when they got pregnant easily. And I didn't want my mum to be sad for me or worry about me. Adam, my husband, was a great support because, as a lifelong optimist, he always believed we'd have our family in the end.

I loathed the hours spent waiting for fertility appointments in gloomy NHS corridors; and the appointments themselves were gruelling and made me feel very vulnerable. If you've ever had an HSG (an hysterosalpingogram, which examines your womb and Fallopian tubes using a dye that shows up when your abdomen is X-rayed), you'll know why I walked out of the examination room when I saw the huge machine I was being asked to lie on, naked from the waist down. Most of the doctors were good at explaining things, and kind, but I still felt like crying at every appointment, just because I felt so sad and powerless. There were times when I couldn't face yet another internal examination (one of the women in the book made me laugh when she said, 'I automatically take off my knickers now as soon as I get into any doctor's examination room').

Hormone tests and cycle monitoring showed my cycle was regular and I was ovulating, but the HSG showed my tubes might be blocked. Two years after I first went to the GP, I was booked in for a laparoscopy (a keyhole operation: a camera is put inside your abdomen via an incision under your tummy button). The surgeon discovered my tubes *were* blocked, and that I had adhesions, bands of tissue stuck to my internal organs, possibly due to a pelvic inflammatory disease that I'd had a few years earlier. Your tubes are so tiny and delicate, they can easily be damaged by infection and by adhesions.

At this point, I was finding it hard to concentrate on anything but my fertility. I could cope pretty well with seeing pregnant friends (of course, this was the exact time lots of friends chose to procreate), but I was beginning to feel bitter towards innocent pregnant strangers in the street. Infertility brought out the nastiest part of me, and altered my perception of the world, so that having a baby became the only thing that counted. I spent hours obsessing over the next test, the next result, preparing for the next treatment, wondering what might make it work or even if I'd magically get pregnant naturally.

The months between NHS appointments dragged on and on. Six months after the first laparoscopy I had another one, this time to clear away the adhesions and attempt to free up my tubes. It didn't work. Another six months later, and I saw another consultant. He looked at my notes, pronounced me a perfect candidate for IVF and referred me on to the NHS IVF waiting list.

I was nervous, as IVF sounded so medical and invasive, but frankly, after three years of blood tests, scans, internals, laparoscopies and waiting, I was relieved to be getting to that next stage. And what was cheering was that although IVF is now used for a whole spectrum of fertility problems – polycystic ovaries, failure to ovulate, endometriosis and male-factor infertility – it was actually invented to bypass malfunctioning tubes like mine.

As the NHS waiting list for IVF was a year in our area at the time, and I was by then 35, we decided we'd better get on with having IVF privately. My mum kindly gave us some money towards it, and we scraped together the rest. I went to see fertility expert Zita West, who talked me through the pros and cons of the many London clinics.

Another six months later, I was at my first appointment at the ARGC – the Assisted Reproduction & Gynaecology Centre in London. But just when I was ready to start my first IVF cycle, a doctor there scanned me and told me that my tubes were full of fluid due to having been blocked. He said that this could stop the IVF working, as the fluid can go into the uterus and prevent the embryo from implanting. Another gynaecologist agreed and said that my tubes and the adhesions around them were probably causing my awful period pains too. So I had another operation – this time to remove my tubes. It was a very final decison to make, and one I have occasionally regretted since. From that point on, IVF would be my only method of ever getting pregnant.

That's when I first found the Fertility Friends website, which has a forum for the ARGC, among other clinics. At first I just read other women's conversations but one day, once I'd finally started IVF, I joined in, asking, 'What does it mean that my left ovary is showing more follicles [the sacs that contain the eggs] than my right?' And, a few days later, 'Does anyone else feel twinges in their ovaries during stimulation? Or get spotting?' I liked that lots of people replied, and everyone supported each other, cheered each other on and commiserated, really knowing what it felt like when things didn't work out. My online fertility buddies were there for me during IVF, at all hours, day or night, ready with a quick boost or supportive comment. One woman who was always helpful on the forum was a GP called Alice, who is still a friend today (and whose story is told in Chapter 12).

It became clear to me that some people who hadn't been through infertility or IVF often didn't 'get it'. Toni (see Chapter 3) explains it like this: 'People who haven't experienced infertility don't understand how it takes over your life, how sad it is that a vision you had of your life has been taken away from you.' It was hard having to explain every step in the IVF process to friends and family, even when they were being loving and wanted to support me. I was lucky because at work, my boss and close workmates were kind too, asking me how things were going every day.

The actual treatment was hardcore and physically demanding. At the ARGC, for the roughly two weeks that you're injecting drugs to stimulate your ovaries to produce eggs, you have a blood test every day at 7 a.m., sometimes two, and scans every other day too. I still can't drive near the blood clinic in Harley Street without feeling my stomach tighten. There was a lot of waiting around for scans and appointments at the clinic too. The waiting room was filled with an air of desperation mixed with camaraderie. People were in awe of Mr Taranissi, the head of the clinic, and talked about 'Mr T.' in reverential tones. I joked later that the chairs shouldn't have been around the edges of the waiting room, but all in lines, as if we were praying to Mr T. Often, I'd chat to a neighbour about our treatments and I'd feel quite lucky, because while I was on my first cycle, others were on their third, even fifth.

I had nine eggs collected in the end (I always think egg collection sounds more like a country pursuit than a surgical procedure). One of these went on to become my gorgeous, now four-year-old, son Patrick. I was nervous while pregnant, even though everything was textbook. And I'm still, to this day, a much more neurotic mother than I would ever have imagined I'd be; taking so long to have a baby changed me, in that way, for ever.

When Patrick was two, we decided to try again with our two remaining frozen embryos. But I didn't get pregnant. I had always said I'd be happy with one child, that I wouldn't have another fresh IVF cycle, but found I couldn't ignore my longing for a second baby, a sibling for Patrick. So we started a new cycle a year later. During a scan leading up to egg collection, I was upset as my eggs weren't developing evenly on each ovary (I was pretty overwrought generally, at the time). The doctor said to me, 'I have women in here who would be very grateful to be in your position.' And I felt quite ashamed.

This time, the result was a biochemical pregnancy. So while at first I did get a positive pregnancy test, for a week my blood levels of beta hCG (the hormone you produce when you're pregnant) stayed the same, and then they started to fall – a sure sign that the pregnancy was over. That was torture. I was bowled over at how hard it hit me. I was already exhausted from the sheer emotional stress and hormone overload, and from juggling appointments with work; I just wanted to curl up under my duvet and hide.

When Adam and I talked about doing IVF one more time, we didn't know if we could go through with it, and we certainly couldn't afford it. Mum asked me, 'If you had enough money, would you have another treatment?' And when she put it like that, I knew I would. 'Never let a lack of money stop you from doing anything,' she said. Her financial help and writing this book (ironically) paid for our next treatment, when I was 41.

That time, we did get pregnant, but, sadly, I lost the pregnancy one day off 16 weeks (that story is in Chapter 20). After a miscarriage, and indeed if you can't get pregnant, the world can seem full of pregnant women and babies, reminding you constantly of what you don't have. Just after my miscarriage, an old friend called out of the blue to say that she was almost the same number of weeks pregnant as I'd been just a few days before; while back at work, a month later, three pregnant women got in the lift with me at the same time. I was a mess for a month and cried every day for the following two.

Now I've accepted I'm the mother of a single child and I do feel extremely lucky for that. At the same time, I'm sad that my son is growing up without a brother or sister. I don't want him to have the whole weight of my expectations, or the whole responsibility of us when we're old. On the upside though, we're a very portable family, Adam and I have lots of time for Patrick and he is a very happy and loved child.

Our mothers and grandmothers didn't have the medical options we have today to 'cure' infertility. Then again, for the most part, they did start trying much younger too, so there wasn't, like there is now, an army of women in their late 30s and early 40s feeling let down by their biology.

Medical science not only gives us hope, but also a huge range of options and decisions, with new breakthroughs being announced every month. Often, however, that also includes the chance to spend an awful lot of money with only a limited chance of success.

What I learned from my own experience, more than anything, is that not getting pregnant is about making decisions. Lots of them. And often, these are involved and technical. For me, first, it was, should I push my GP to refer me for investigations after a year of trying or wait another six months? Then it was which IVF clinic is best – should I go to a clinic that has slightly better results, or one that provides more personal attention, or one that's closer to home? Even as a health journalist, the amount of information that's out there seemed overwhelming. Every decision was emotionally charged, as every choice could in theory make the difference between having the longed-for baby – and not. The final decision that my husband and I had to make was: is it time to stop treatment? Financially, it was just about impossible for us to continue, but emotionally, I reasoned, did I really want to put all of us – including Patrick – on to the IVF rollercoaster again when our chance of success was so low?

Every woman in this book has had to make these kinds of decisions, and has made them in her own way. Their stories are not supposed to be a practical guide – there are plenty of other books out there fulfilling that need (you'll find recommendations at the end of each chapter and in the Further reading section on page 311). Rather, they are intended to show you what others have done in the situation that you are in, what it felt like for them and how they made their decisions along the way.

My day job is Health Editor of *Red* magazine, and the inspiration for the book came from *Red*'s Annual National Fertility Report. I wrote it in the period from a few months before my final IVF cycle to a few months after the miscarriage.

All the women I interviewed taught me something that helped me in my final cycle, or that has stayed with me. For example, Amanda (see Chapter 1), showed me that you can choose to see IVF failure as a nightmare or you can view it as a learning experience for the next cycle. Oona (see Chapter 18), taught me to accept that, during fertility treatment, it's normal for your emotions to be overwhelming. And lastly, Sinead (Chapter 9) helped me realise that when you don't get what you want, you should still be thankful for what you do have.

Hopefully, this book will show that for every desperate moment, for every heart-breaking test result and for every difficult decision you face, someone else has probably been there before you. And she's here – and happy – to tell her story.

Why I had IVF

• • • • • • • • • • • • •

'I was ovulating, but not getting pregnant.
And I desperately wanted to know why.
It was so frustrating.'

'All babies are miracles, but IVF babies are
real miracles.'

'My mantra was: "As long as there's one egg,
I can get pregnant."'

'After three IUIs in four months, I started
pushing the doctors to recommend IVF because
the success rates are so much better than IUI.'

'When I looked at him, he was the person whose
biological children I wanted. I wanted a mini
Nick running around, not to have to think about
using somebody else's sperm.'

Polycystic ovaries stopped me ovulating

• • • • • • • • • • • •

'The symptoms of PCOS all directly attack your femininity: facial hair, spots, weight gain. But the worst one of all is lack of periods and the resulting infertility,' says Theresa Cheung, co-author of the book *PCOS and Your Fertility*, who herself underwent medical treatment to conceive her two children. 'Getting pregnant felt like something I should have been able to do as a woman. It seemed so easy for other people. But I had to accept that it wasn't going to happen for me naturally, that I needed medical help,' she says.

As the most common hormonal disorder for women, affecting up to 10 per cent, PCOS (polycystic ovary syndrome) is a major cause of fertility problems. As you may know, with PCOS it's not that you're not producing eggs, it's that you don't actually ovulate, which leaves your ovaries filled with follicles that have failed to launch – the so-called 'cysts'. 'The hormonal environment in the ovaries isn't conducive to ovulation,' explains Mr Tarek El-Toukhy, Consultant and

Honorary Lecturer in Reproductive Medicine and Surgery at Guy's and St Thomas' Hospital NHS Foundation Trust.

It's now generally agreed that lifestyle is key for controlling PCOS symptoms, and healthy living can help to regulate your cycle. 'Weight loss, if the patient is overweight, and exercise can both decrease the intensity of polycystic ovaries, and we see a lot of success just by doing this,' says Mr El-Toukhy. Theresa agrees: 'My symptoms – including a lack of periods – come back if I'm not taking care of myself by eating badly or not exercising enough.'

If you have PCOS, you'll probably have had months, possibly years, of medical treatment by the time you reach an IVF clinic, usually starting with a drug treatment: one to induce ovulation, such as clomiphene (Clomid), and/or metformin, a drug used to treat diabetes. If this doesn't work, the next line of attack is often an operation called ovarian drilling (this is exactly as it sounds). 'We don't know precisely how this operation works, but it could be related to the release of chemical substances within the tissue of the ovary, contributing to changes in the local hormonal environment and stimulating ovulation,' says Mr El-Toukhy. Next comes IUI (intrauterine insemination – where sperm is put into the uterus around the time of ovulation), using the same ovary-stimulating drugs as IVF and, finally, IVF (although a lot of women choose to go straight from Clomid to IVF).

• • • • • • • • •

Amanda, 35, a public relations director from London, only found out she had PCOS when she came off the Pill. When ovulation-inducing drugs didn't work, she started IVF.

I had no idea that I had polycystic ovaries until my weight ballooned when I stopped taking the Pill. I went from a size 10/12 to a size 16 in a matter of months. I'd been on the Pill since I was 17, when I first got together with Adam. By my late 20s, I wasn't happy that I'd been taking it for so long and Adam and I were about to get married, so I came off it.

Around six months after the wedding, I decided to see a doctor and get myself checked out because of the weight I'd gained and the fact that my periods had become so irregular too. That's when I was diagnosed with PCOS.

At the time, we weren't trying to get pregnant, but we weren't being too careful either. For contraception, we were simply avoiding sex on the days I assumed I was ovulating. Once I was diagnosed with PCOS, it turned out that my actual cycle was so irregular, I'd been avoiding the wrong days. So, in theory, I should have got pregnant and we had, in a way, been trying for eight months with no success.

I started to use an ovulation kit, but it didn't really work because I had such an erratic cycle. When I was monitored to see how often I was ovulating, there was no rhythm or reason to my cycle: sometimes I'd ovulate every two months, sometimes every four. Because I was ovulating so rarely, I realised we only really had around four chances a year to get pregnant. So when I was prescribed clomiphene (Clomid), a drug to make me ovulate, I was quite optimistic – you hear a lot of miracle stories about Clomid.

The first month I took it, scans showed I didn't ovulate. So the next month, the consultant doubled my dose. You do hear bad things about Clomid too, how it can give you mood swings, but luckily I wasn't affected. This time I did respond and, amazingly, I got pregnant.

A couple of weeks later, on my birthday, I suddenly felt very hormonal, and found myself crying for no reason. I tentatively put it down to being pregnant. Later that day, we went out for a family lunch. I felt some cramping then, during the meal, I started bleeding. When we'd finished eating, I told everyone we were going shopping but, in fact, Adam and I went to the hospital.

There, the nurse asked me to do a urine sample for a pregnancy test, then told me I was no longer pregnant. I came home and cried all night, devastated.

With my sister's first baby due, my parents flew off to Hong Kong to visit her the next day, while I went back to my gynaecologist for a check-up. Just as I'd parked outside his surgery in Harley Street, my phone rang. It was my brother-in-law, calling from Hong Kong, to tell me I had a nephew. That hurt. I was genuinely happy for my sister and him but, at the same time, I felt sad and a real sense of loss for Adam and me.

The gynaecologist said that if I wanted, I could carry on with Clomid in my next cycle without a break. With hindsight, I can see I should have taken a couple of months to get over what had happened, both physically and emotionally. I felt sad for a long time. What did help was telling myself that there was a reason the pregnancy hadn't continued, that the baby most likely wasn't chromosomally right.

Ideally, you're only supposed to take Clomid for six months, but I ended up on it for eight. I didn't want to give up. I thought it was supposed to be a miracle drug, so I couldn't understand why it wasn't working for me. I was ovulating, but not getting pregnant. And I desperately wanted to know why. It was so frustrating.

I was referred to another private consultant, who took me off Clomid and put me on a drug called metformin. This helps to control blood-sugar levels, which can be high in PCOS, and can regulate your cycle so you start ovulating. She explained that it would take a couple of months to work, and if metformin alone didn't make me ovulate, I could combine it with Clomid. If I didn't get pregnant, she explained, the next step would be IUI.

As someone who's extremely organised and used to being in control, those months of waiting for the metformin to work were hard for me. I kept thinking: friends are getting pregnant with their second babies and I'm struggling to fall pregnant with my first. And I was conscious that I'd be even older if and when I had a second child. The pregnancy I'd lost was still very much on my mind, and it was coming up to the due date. It felt like time was running away and there was nothing I could do about it. The one positive sign was that the metformin was helping me lose weight.

Two cycles of metformin and Clomid together didn't get me pregnant, so we started IUI. That ramped up the stress levels. We were spending nearly £1000 a cycle and I was trying to fit in all the appointments with work, taking cabs to the clinic in lunch breaks because I was so busy.

The actual procedure itself wasn't fun either. The sperm transfer had to be done with a full bladder, and waiting for my turn was very uncomfortable. I know being stressed probably didn't stop the IUI from working, but it certainly didn't make it very pleasurable. Every time IUI didn't work, we booked in for another round. Looking back, I can see we should have stopped after two or three times but we were advised to keep going. It was like groundhog day: every month, I'd find myself back at the clinic. Finally, Adam and I decided our fifth IUI would be our last, and it was time for IVF.

I was referred to Guy's and St Thomas'. We had all the standard tests and we were surprised to hear that Adam's sperm count had dropped, never previously a problem. The embryologists recommended that once I'd had my eggs collected, they should be fertilised with ICSI (intracytoplasmic sperm injection – where a single sperm is injected into each egg), explaining it would give us the best chance of fertilisation.

The staff, who were friendly and professional, put us at our ease, and made us both feel confident. The only thing that made me feel a bit sick was the thought of injecting myself with the ovary-stimulating drugs – I'm not good with needles or inflicting pain on myself. So Adam said he'd do them.

We had to do our first injection at a friend's wedding – in a Portaloo, of all places. Holding the little bag of needles and drugs, we were trying to stay calm when someone knocked on the door. The injections are dispensed by a type of pen, and we'd been told to hold it down for five seconds. But because we were so paranoid, we counted out loud to 10, just to be sure. Goodness knows what the person waiting for the loo must have thought!

I dealt with IVF by going through the motions quite mechanically. Fortunately, the drugs didn't affect my mood or emotions, so I was able to carry on with life as normally and unemotionally as possible. But, doing my last injection, I accidentally knocked the glass vial on to the ground and it smashed. So at 8 p.m., we had the panic of trying to get a replacement. Luckily, the clinic said they could fax a prescription to a pharmacy near us. But it took ages to find one that stocked the right drug, would accept a faxed prescription and was still open at what was by then 9.30 p.m. Looking back, it was farcical, but at the time, it felt like a disaster.

When it came to the day of egg collection, we were pleased to get 12 eggs. We felt as if we'd got over the first big hurdle. Three days later, we had nine good embryos and the choice of putting one or two back. We automatically said two, as we wanted our chances to be as good as possible. Once the embryos were in, I felt that there was nothing more I could do. It was in the lap of the gods.

A week after transfer, we took the Eurostar to a family wedding in Paris. When we arrived, I tried on my outfit – a black A-line skirt in a size 12 and a matching top – but I couldn't do the zip up as my belly had expanded so much since I'd left London. I had to go shopping for new clothes and borrow a pair of my sister's maternity tights (she was by then pregnant with her second child). I looked five months pregnant and a man in Galleries Lafayette actually gave me a chair because he thought I needed a break!

At the wedding, I felt uncomfortable because I thought people would assume I was pregnant too. I knew the bloating was probably caused by mild OHSS (ovarian hyperstimulation syndrome), which I'd been warned about by the clinic. The main advice is to drink a lot of water, so I was going to the loo all the time. I could hardly move, I didn't dance, and I felt huge. Towards the end of the evening, my sides started hurting too and I began to feel really uncomfortable and knackered.

When we got back from Paris, I called the clinic, and told them about my bloating. They asked me to come in, in case they needed to put in a drain to take out the excess fluid that builds up with OHSS. The first thing the nurse asked was if I'd done my pregnancy test. I said no, because I thought I wasn't due to take it for another two days. And she said, 'No, you were supposed to take it yesterday!' How the hell had I got my test date wrong? Probably because I'd been so determined to go on with normal life, and not think about IVF, that I'd pushed it to the back of my mind.

In shock and on autopilot, I went to the toilet and peed on the test stick. I didn't even look at it. In my mind, I wanted to give the test to the nurse, go home and for her to call me with the result. As I passed the test to her, a faint line on it caught my eye. I said, 'Oh, I guess that means the treatment didn't work; there's only a faint line.' She said, 'Actually, that means you *are* pregnant.'

I couldn't believe it. I was elated, but made myself stay calm as I knew it was early days for the pregnancy. I went through the rest of the examination in a daze. Luckily, I didn't need any treatment for the OHSS, and was just told to drink more water.

I called Adam, told him that the OHSS wasn't serious and rambled on about my appointment before saying casually, 'Oh, by the way, I'm pregnant'. He was ecstatic, of course. We decided not to tell anyone for a while, because of losing the previous pregnancy and the fact that this one was still so new.

Two weeks later, I started bleeding at work. It's just not fair, I thought. It's happening again. Adam called NHS Direct, who told us to go to A & E. After waiting for hours, we finally persuaded the doctor to do a scan. Incredibly, we saw one heartbeat, and that was a huge relief. There was another sac, but it looked like a dark circle with nothing in it. The doctor said, 'There's one heartbeat, but it looks as if the other embryo didn't make it.'

That was the first time that the idea of twins had crossed either of our minds. I actually felt a loss for the second twin, thinking that it had grown inside me for a few weeks. But, as Adam said, we should be very grateful for our one healthy heartbeat. My mum, who has a medical background, said it was probably a good thing that we'd ended up with one, as twins can be such a difficult pregnancy, and often one or both of the babies is sickly or they're premature. Everyone put a positive spin on the situation but, for me, it was still bittersweet.

Then, at our first official scan at the IVF clinic, at eight weeks, just as I was telling the doctor we'd only seen one heartbeat, she said, 'Well, now you've got two'. I practically fell off the bed. She explained that the heartbeat comes between six and eight weeks of pregnancy, and the first scan was probably too early. We were shocked, but also delighted.

Even though I was only a couple of months pregnant, my stomach was very big, so I told people at work that I had something wrong with my digestion (I'd had digestive problems in the past). It wasn't until after the 12-week scan, when we found out that both babies were healthy, that we finally felt confident enough to share our news. But, at 15 weeks, I suddenly started bleeding again. I kept thinking: I don't want to lose one, they come as a pair, but, despite feeling well, I could only assume we'd lost one or both babies, as there was so much blood.

At A & E, after several examinations by different doctors, none of whom could find anything wrong with the pregnancy, it was discovered that I had a burst polyp – a little growth on my cervix – and that this was what had bled. The doctor was very kind and understanding and I'll always remember him saying to me: 'All babies are miracles, but IVF babies are real miracles.'

For the rest of the pregnancy, I had scans every two or three weeks, which made me feel safe. Nathan and Dylan were born healthy, by C-section, exactly a month early (they did go into special care for two weeks because they couldn't yet feed). After they were born, all thoughts of Clomid, IUI and IVF disappeared. It's no longer relevant to me how the boys were conceived. All that matters is that we have two healthy, lovely children.

Q: WERE YOU OFFERED ANY OTHER TREATMENTS FOR PCOS?

After we decided to stop having IUI, I did see a consultant who recommended a procedure called ovarian drilling, where a surgeon makes holes in your ovaries in order to restart your cycle. I did consider it, even went on the waiting list, but it seemed very extreme. I thought of it as a last resort, if IVF didn't work.

Q: HOW ARE YOUR PCOS SYMPTOMS NOW?

The boys were born in January and I was thin within a couple of months, but by June of that year, I had put on loads of weight again. I could also see that I was a little more hairy too. Even though metformin had suited me so well, and the doctors were happy for me to go back on it, I didn't want to take it. I didn't like the idea of being on medication for ever. And I didn't think, with the babies, I'd remember to take it three times a day, in any case. I kept thinking: maybe the symptoms will calm down or I'll eat less. When the twins were three, I decided to go back on metformin. It has made a difference – I'm definitely less hungry and I'm down to a size 10/12 again.

Q: DID YOU TELL PEOPLE WHILE YOU WERE HAVING IVF?

I was quite happy to tell some people about our fertility treatment, but not everyone. I worked up until twenty-nine weeks; one of my final tasks was organising a celebrity event. Everyone there kept saying to me, 'Oh my God, you're massive,' assuming I was about to drop there and then. So I had to explain it was a twin pregnancy, and the inevitable next question was always, 'Oh, have you got twins in the family?' and, 'Are they identical?' When people ask if there are twins in the family, I think what they're really saying is, 'Was it IVF?' But, to be honest, I'm not embarrassed by it. I usually say simply that it was fertility treatment – most people don't ask for details.

I'm also asked, 'What are you going to tell the children about how they were conceived?' But I don't think they're going to care about the actual mechanism of conception, especially these days. I was making dinner the other day, stirring something, and Dylan said, 'Is that how you made us?' He knew that he and Nathan had been in my stomach, and assumed they must have got there the same way as food! If we'd used donor sperm or eggs, I think it would be different, as then it's a question of genetics.

Q: WHAT WILL YOU DO WITH YOUR FROZEN EMBRYOS?

We've got seven embryos frozen from our treatment. Recently, I got a letter saying that they're about to reach their five-year deadline, and we have to decide what to do with them. We're not going to use them ourselves, as we don't want any more children. We're still having a debate about what to do with them. If it was just my eggs, I could donate them to someone who needs them. But I'm not comfortable doing that with embryos, as they are, theoretically, full siblings to Nathan and Dylan. If I did, I might start thinking every child I see on the street is genetically ours. I would like to give them to medical research, as for me it's important to give back, but Adam isn't keen as he doesn't want them to be prodded and experimented on. He'd rather let them be destroyed. I think I'll probably win the argument in the end, but it might take a while.

Q: WHAT'S YOUR BEST ADVICE FOR ANYONE DOING IVF?

You need to keep calm. I'm sure that part of the reason why IVF worked for us is that we're quite calm people. And I made sure I stayed that way. My belief is, only worry about things when you absolutely need to.

Also, try to be positive and don't think about it not working. Try to go about your normal daily life and don't let everything be about IVF. Just before I had IVF, I met a woman who'd had multiple cycles of IVF and had made some extreme life changes she thought would help it work. She was on a strict organic diet, not using foil or plastic on her food and avoiding microwaved food. But I knew that wouldn't have suited me. I believed that the more changes I made away from my normal life, the more I would have been setting myself up for disappointment had IVF failed.

The hard thing, when you're having fertility problems, is when your friends are falling pregnant around you – especially, I found, when they are having their second. But you have to be positive and think: their second won't take away my first.

Q: WHO WAS YOUR SUPPORT SYSTEM?

I had my best friends, my parents and, of course, my husband Adam, although, ironically, I probably spoke to him about it less, as I didn't want it to be all-consuming for us. After a while, Adam's attitude was sometimes, 'Do we really need to talk about this again?' He always believed it would happen for us. And, as a man, he wasn't as conscious of my biological clock, so he didn't mind if it happened straight away or in a year.

• • • • • • • • •

Difficult though it is to live with the symptoms of PCOS, the good news is that the majority of women who have it and want to get pregnant, do so. But that doesn't mean it isn't a hard slog to get to that point.

For excess weight associated with PCOS, some women swear by the GI diet: 'Many nutritionists, dietitians, and women with PCOS believe the lower sugar and lower refined carbohydrates in the GI diet really work, by reducing insulin resistance and keeping hunger pangs at bay,' explains Colette Harris, co-author of *PCOS and Your Fertility* (Hay House) and *The Ultimate PCOS Handbook* (Thorsons). 'The basis of the diet is more protein, more fibre and less sugar,' she says. And while there's no consensus on how often or how hard you should exercise, she recommends some exercise every day, even if it's just gardening or brisk walking.

If you are keen to explore complementary treatment for PCOS, a Swedish study from 2010,[1] where women had 16 weeks of electroacupuncture (where the needles are linked up to a minimal electric current) had more periods as a result. Fertility acupuncturist Emma Cannon (emmacannon. co.uk) says that most of her clients find their cycles return after one to two months of acupuncture.

And there's more good news: a study published in 2010 from the Shahid Beheshti University in Iran[2] compared the AMH blood levels (anti-Müllerian hormone – a marker of fertility) of women with PCOS and those without, and found that AMH declined to menopausal levels on average two years later in women with PCOS, which means they have a better chance of conceiving at a slightly older age[3].

Finally, Verity, the PCOS charity, runs conferences with expert speakers (verity-pcos.org.uk); you do need to be a member, but they can keep you up to speed on all the latest research. You can download previous conference speeches at the website of PCOS-UK, the education arm of Verity (pcos-uk.org.uk).

My partner had no sperm

• • • • • • • • • • •

'W hen a man finds out that he's subfertile, it can be a huge knock. Thinking he might not be a father can change how he feels about himself,' says fertility coach, Anya Sizer.

A low or even a zero sperm count doesn't mean a man can't be a father, though. 'There is a range of sperm counts in men, some have lots, some very few,' says Dr Allan Pacey, Senior Lecturer in Andrology at the University of Sheffield. 'And the definition of healthy sperm count recently went down from 20 million per millilitre to 15 million. At that level, a man should be able to become a father within a year. But you can be "abnormal" by that definition and manage it in, for example, two years.'

Male fertility treatment has seen the biggest technological advances in the past 10 years. 'We don't have any magic pills to stimulate men to produce more sperm. What we do have are ways of extracting sperm or doing the best we can with the sperm that we can get,' says Dr Pacey. By using intracytoplasmic sperm injection, or ICSI, embryologists can now fertilise an egg with a single sperm.

Even if tests show zero sperm in a man's ejaculate, there are several surgical techniques that can extract sperm, when previously a man would have had to use a donor to have a family. 'Finding nothing in ejaculate is unfortunate,' says Dr Pacey, 'but it doesn't necessarily mean that a man's testicles aren't producing any sperm, just that they're not making it out in the ejaculate or they haven't been seen in the lab. When we look at ejaculate, usually several millilitres of fluid, it's impossible to look in every single bit of it. Theoretically, there could still be several thousand sperm in there, when we see nothing.'

The major factors that affect sperm count and/or quality are genetics (including having undescended testicles at birth), trauma, chemotherapy and vasectomy. The surgery of choice if there's a blockage, for example after vasectomy, is aspiration via a needle, usually taken out of the tube which carries sperm from the testes to the penis (PESA – percutaneous epididymal sperm aspiration), but sometimes from the testicle itself (TESA – testicular sperm aspiration). These are procedures that are performed every day.

My dad had a vasectomy over 20 years ago, which meant he couldn't have it reversed when he wanted to have a child in his 60s. So he had PESA to help conceive his now toddler daughter: 'I had a full anaesthetic but I was only out for thirty minutes. There was no pain or bruising afterwards; the only slightly embarrassing part was that the nurse who helped with the op was so chatty!'

'After a vasectomy, there's usually a hundred per cent success rate at getting sperm surgically. These men were obviously fertile in the first place,' says Dr Pacey. But, he explains, 'With a man whose fertility has been affected by chemotherapy, the success rate is perhaps about forty per cent.' These men, or those who had undescended testicles at birth, may need to have an operation called TESE (testicular sperm extraction), where tissue is removed from the testicles, then dissected to find any sperm.

There are a lot of other factors affecting sperm quality and quantity too. These include sexually transmitted infections ('In my lab's last study, thirteen per cent of men referred by their GP for fertility tests had chlamydia and didn't know it,' says Dr Pacey), flu or any illness with a temperature, prescription medicines including some SSRI antidepressants and anabolic steroids, sitting down a lot (for example, men who drive a car for more than two hours a day), smoking, over-drinking, working with various chemicals (glycol ethers, in paint, glues, dry cleaning fluids) and long exposure to lead in petrol or exhaust fumes.

Of course, even once you have the sperm, pregnancy isn't guaranteed, as Ella, whose story is below, found out, because to do ICSI, you're relying on the success of IVF.

• • • • • • • • •

Ella, 37, a marketing manager from Bristol, and her husband Nick were told that he had a zero sperm count.

Nick was at the airport with a group of his friends, about to go away on a boys' weekend to Berlin, when he got the call to say he wasn't producing any sperm. He'd had the test done at our local hospital, and when the nurse called him to give him the results, he was sitting in the bar, drinking with his mates. To be in that testosterone-fuelled environment, then be told you have no sperm count and, therefore, no chance of fathering a baby seemed the ultimate irony. He had half expected it, but it was still a shock. His very worst fears had turned out to be true.

Nick had been concerned about his fertility ever since his early teens. That's when he'd found out that when he was born, his testes were still inside his body – 'undescended'. He did have an operation to correct it, but not until he was six years old. Nowadays, doctors think it's best to do that operation as early as possible, as it's thought that high temperatures inside the body may affect sperm production later in life. The actual operation may do so too.

Nick told me about the operation within a couple of weeks of us starting to get serious, so I knew it was important to him. Without him telling me, I'd never have known he'd had it; as an adult, the only sign was a tiny scar on each side of his testes.

Once we'd got the news he was producing zero sperm, my first thought was to find a solution. We asked to be referred to a urologist (a specialist who deals with male parts), but he told us the same thing as our GP: that our options were now sperm donation or adoption. He also did some blood tests, which confirmed that Nick wasn't producing any sperm, despite the appearance that things were working normally. It was our first encounter with a specialist, and I was shocked at how, for him, it was an everyday job. Considering he was telling us our future, he seemed quite offhand – he even answered the phone in the middle of our consultation and chatted for 10 minutes. He was so used to dealing with fertility issues, it wasn't a big deal to him, but it was our life.

Because Nick had worried about not being fertile for so long, then had had his worst nightmare confirmed, it was pretty hard to find the right way to help him. It felt as if I was treading on eggshells. The hardest part was that it had happened to him when he was little, and so he had had no control over it. It wasn't as if he'd taken steroids or even that he'd had cancer or an accident. I know he was thinking: why me?

I was devastated too. We'd just got married but, potentially, I was facing not being able to have his child. That was a really sad prospect. Part of getting married was wanting to create a family together. When I looked at him, he was the person whose biological children I wanted. I wanted a mini Nick running around, not to have to think about using somebody else's sperm. So while I was trying to be strong for him, I was trying to deal with my own emotions too.

But I'm a very persistent person, so we went back for a second appointment to ask if there were any other tests we could do. The specialist said there was one option – an operation called TESE, where incisions are made in the testes, at the top and bottom, some of the sperm-producing tissue is removed, then whatever sperm is found in it is retrieved and frozen. I'd have to have IVF to produce eggs, then Nick's sperm would be thawed and injected into my eggs, using the ICSI technique.

The specialist told us that some clinics and hospitals are more experienced and better than others at TESE, so I asked him the very best place to have the operation. He mentioned a clinic in Brussels, where ICSI was actually pioneered.

Nick and I discussed whether or not to go ahead and decided that we didn't have much to lose. If the operation didn't work, at least we would have done everything we could to have our own biological child. We didn't feel we could move on to thinking about donor sperm or adoption until we knew that.

So, a few weeks later, we booked our flights to Brussels. The clinic there was quite a culture shock after what we'd seen of British hospitals. It was modern in its design and high-tech. The staff were very welcoming and professional. There was no language problem because we were assigned an English-speaking counsellor, and she arranged and attended all our appointments and was our point of contact throughout the whole process.

When we met with our consultant, he made us feel comfortable too. He assured us that a lot of couples were in our situation, and said that Nick was a suitable candidate for the operation. He explained that there would be an embry-ologist in the operating theatre with a microscope, and as soon as the tissue was removed, he or she would check the sample for sperm immediately, and freeze whatever was found. He also said that if they didn't find any sperm during the operation, the clinic would help us to move on to other options.

That night, we went out for dinner in Brussels. We'd decided to spend some of the money we'd saved for treat-ment on dinner, a nice hotel and some sightseeing. It was April, and it was warm, so we ate outside in Brussels' famous and very beautiful historic square, Grand-Place. Being away from home together felt very special. Some of the usual stresses disappeared and it gave us time to talk – I think Nick was the most open he's ever been.

We were put on the waiting list at the Brussels clinic, but amazingly the counsellor called the next day to say they'd had a cancellation for two weeks later. So we booked in.

Once we got home, however, we began to get nervous. It's obviously not great for a guy to have his bits sliced up, and we had also been warned there was a small risk his testoster-one levels could drop after the operation, so he'd have to be on hormone replacement therapy, and the drop would put him at risk of osteoporosis too.

The more I read up, the more I worried. I lost my dad when I was fifteen and since then I've had a phobia of hospitals. I got completely carried away, thinking: Nick and I have only been married six months; will I lose him too?

That's where the counsellor came into her own. She told us on the phone that the clinic did the same operation every single day. And she explained that some men do have a tiny drop in hormones after surgery, but that it usually only lasts for around a year. I was vocal about my fears to Nick, but he stayed level-headed. He said the operation didn't scare him, and that it was very important for him to know if he could father a child or not.

Two weeks later, we were back in Brussels. The night before the operation, I had to help Nick remove the hair from his bits using cream. I know a lot of men do shave or wax now, but I'm not sure many of them use Immac! It was a really girly scented one too, and that made it even funnier. Nick made me swear never to tell his mates.

On the morning of the operation, I was so nervous that I hurried us too much, and we arrived at the hospital an hour early, at 6.30 a.m. I didn't want to be teary in front of Nick, but I was feeling very emotional. I was terrified he wouldn't come round from the operation. He, of course, was absolutely fine, being his usual self and joking around when they gave him some unattractive paper pants to put on.

We waited in a room with a Dutch couple who were having the same operation. Luckily, we were going first. Nick was put on the bed to go to theatre at 8 a.m. He's quite a big muscular guy, and when he lay down, the trolley started to collapse. I couldn't help but laugh.

As soon as they took Nick off to theatre, I started crying. I was so worried. I kept thinking that making a baby is supposed to be a special experience, not a medical one. I felt lonely, knowing he was under anaesthetic, and that the outcome would decide if we could have children or not. I thought he was so brave to have the operation. A tiny bit of me was hopeful, but I kept talking myself out of it because I didn't want to be let down if it didn't work.

It only took a couple of hours for Nick to come round after surgery, but it felt like for ever. When he was wheeled into the recovery room, he was still high, so he was joking around a bit, telling me how pretty the nurses were. I was pleased he was positive, but he was also quite groggy and it was unnerving to see him not being himself.

A nurse came in and said, 'I hear it's good news.' I said, 'Oh no, I don't think so.' I was so convinced it wouldn't be. But the nurse went on, 'No, they looked at the tissue in theatre and they found sperm.'

Nick went to sleep at that point, and I was sure she had confused our results with the Dutch couple's. But an hour or so later, our specialist came in and gave us both a massive hug. He said they'd found plenty of sperm; on one side, they hadn't found anything (the original operation to bring down the testicles had, apparently, been botched), but on the other, they'd managed to extract twelve straws. Each straw is a vial the size of a match, and you only need one to have ICSI. We still had quite a lot to do before we could have a baby, but we were on our way.

While we were hugging and laughing with relief, the Dutch couple had found out they had a negative result. We could hear the woman crying through the curtains around her partner's bed, and we really felt for them. It so easily could have been us.

As we left the clinic later that afternoon, Nick wasn't in any pain, but he was walking like John Wayne, as if he'd just got off a horse, which made us laugh. Amazingly, the swelling went down fast after the first day, and after a week or so, the stitches had dissolved; after two weeks the wounds were completely healed. The surgeon had gone in through the same incisions that had been made when Nick was a child, so there were no new scars. We were so impressed and grateful; I even called the surgeon to say what a great job he'd done.

I wanted to crack on with my part of the treatment to keep the momentum going. Scans and blood tests at the clinic showed that I was ovulating and producing lots of eggs, so I could start the injections to stimulate my ovaries a few weeks later. The counsellor showed me how to do the injections on an orange, and I soon got over my needle phobia.

It was quite complicated to be treated abroad: I was being monitored at a clinic near home, who would fax my results to work, then I'd fax them on to Brussels. Then Brussels would call me to say if I should change my drug dosage. Once the follicles were a certain size, I did the injection to make me ovulate, and we got on the Eurostar the next morning. It was scary, knowing I was about to release all my eggs, and I spent the whole journey hoping we'd get to Brussels on time.

I was nervous about the egg-collection procedure, but it helped that Nick had already had an operation. He was very supportive, though I could tell he hated that I was having to go through so much.

In the morning – roughly 36 hours after my final injection – I was wheeled into the same operating theatre where Nick had had his surgery a few weeks before. Egg collection is done under local anaesthetic at that clinic, so I had an injection in my bottom. But I don't think it worked, as once they started doing the actual egg retrieval, via a needle through my vagina, I felt everything. I'm normally quite good with pain, but I was in agony. The only way I can describe it is like someone pushing a red-hot needle into your lower tummy, then feeling something being sucked out. Because I'd never had it done before, I assumed this was how it was meant to be, so when the nurse asked me if I was ok, I kept saying I was fine. For the first four or five eggs, I thought I could cope, but then the pain got too much and the anaesthetist put something in my drip, which helped a bit.

In all, they collected 18 eggs, and the whole process took half an hour. When I was wheeled into recovery, I told Nick how horrific it had been. I couldn't move as I was in so much pain. But we had good news almost straight away: 16 out of the 18 eggs were viable.

Then we were on to the next worry: would Nick's sperm survive defrosting? It did, but the clinic don't give out any more information about fertilisation, so we had to endure three days without news of the embryos. We were staying in a nice hotel which helped take our minds off what was happening at the clinic, but it was a nerve-wracking time.

On day three, we were having breakfast, when the counsellor called to say they'd like to do the transfer in two hours. We were very excited and phoned our families to say that it was finally going ahead. I felt much happier about going into the theatre with Nick holding my hand this time.

But once we got to the clinic, there was bad news. Of the 18 eggs, only three had actually fertilised and only one was still alive at day three. We told each other that we only needed one, that it could still work, but the quality of the embryo wasn't that great, and we were disappointed. All that effort and stress, all those injections, and we were left with a single, solitary hope.

After transfer, I rested in bed at the hotel for three days, as I felt that would give it the best chance of working, then we took the Eurostar home. The two-week wait was hard; with every tweak and sensation, I couldn't help questioning if I was pregnant or not. Then, the day before the end of the two-week wait, I was about to go out to my sister's birthday party, when I got my period. Even when you're trying to get pregnant naturally and you get your period, it feels as if you're losing something. But this time, that feeling was much more brutal.

Somewhere, I knew there was a little embryo that hadn't taken. We'd had mainly good news until this point, so it took us a while to realise that, this time, it really was bad news.

I wanted to try again straight away, but when I rang the clinic, they advised us to wait three months, to give my body time to settle down. They were really encouraging; they said we should think of our first go as a trial, and that we had loads of sperm left.

I think taking that break was sensible, even though it felt as if we were back to square one. That was our lowest point. I needed to keep talking about it, but Nick was happy to talk about it just once or twice, then move on.

We hadn't lived a normal life for ages, so we tried to spend time together, and see friends and family. There were a lot of weddings that summer. It was hard because we hadn't told anyone we were having treatment, and people kept asking us when we were starting a family. At home afterwards, I'd always end up in tears.

The second treatment cycle was pretty much the same as the first: 16 eggs but, in the end, only one embryo was viable. It was easier, as I knew about the injections and all the procedures. In the end, we were unlucky again. I found out I wasn't pregnant when I went to the loo at a friend's wedding and I'd got my period. I went out and had a glass of champagne, because I could. I felt awful.

The next morning, lying in bed, I was idly Googling IVF, and I put in 'best results'. The ARGC in London came up. Nick had wanted to wait for few months for our next treatment, but I was impatient. I managed to get an appointment for a few weeks later, and took the train to London.

I was expecting a grand Harley Street set-up, but the ARGC is pretty well worn. The doctor we saw was very helpful and easy to talk to. Pricewise, I knew it was more expensive than some other UK clinics, as there are a lot of extras (for example, daily blood tests), but then travelling to Brussels hadn't been cheap either.

The doctor recommended I have a hysteroscopy – an operation where the doctors look inside your womb using a camera inserted via your vagina – which, he said, may help increase the chances of success. I had to be monitored for a month too, so we couldn't start the actual treatment for a couple of months.

In the meantime, I went part-time at work, as working full-time and doing IVF had become too stressful. I borrowed a flat in London, as I had to have daily blood tests and go into the clinic for scans and drugs too. The nurses and staff were very kind and, through talking to the other women I met there, I learned that everyone seemed to be on different drugs and dosages, so I was confident that I was getting treatment personalised to me.

The day of egg collection and fertilisation was nail-biting. We had arranged for Nick's sperm to come over by courier from Brussels, but the flight was delayed. Nick had to be in the clinic early, ready to have another operation, just in case the sperm didn't arrive or hadn't survived.

To my huge relief, egg collection at the ARGC is done under general anaesthetic, so I didn't feel a thing. When I woke up, the nurses were laughing. I asked if everything was ok, and they said, 'Yes – we're now calling you the eighty-egg girl!' Apparently, in my half-awake state, I'd asked a nurse how many eggs they'd collected, and, though she'd said 18, I'd thought she said 80, and repeated it.

It took the embryologists an hour to find viable sperm in the straws. In the end, they found enough and did ICSI on my eggs. Out of the 18 eggs, this time 16 fertilised. By day three, we still had eight good embryos, so they said we should hold off until day five, when the embryos would reach blastocyst stage (an advanced stage of development); this would allow

them to choose those that had the best chance of implantation. On day five, they called us and said, 'Actually, we still
can't choose between them, as they're all looking good, so
we're going to wait until day six.' We had two good-quality
blastocysts to put in that day. Sadly, the others had started to
die away, so we had none to freeze.

I was really churned up. It felt like we'd reached the end
of a big journey and I couldn't work out what we'd do next if
I didn't get pregnant. Before embryo transfer, I asked if I
could see the embryos, but the doctor, Mr Taranissi, said that
too much movement can be traumatic for them, and that he
preferred to put them straight in. After transfer, he left us
alone for half an hour, saying, 'This is your moment to be
together.'

I felt so full of emotion. I said to Nick that I could feel it
working. He told me not to be silly, that it was far too early,
but I really did feel positive. When it was time to stand up, I
was scared. But the embryologist reassured me with a really
clever image. He described the womb lining as being like the
bread of a jam sandwich, so the embryos couldn't fall out. I
still spent the journey back home the next day with my feet
up on the dashboard, though. I must have looked like Lady
Muck, the back seat crammed with bags from my month
spent shopping in London, and the seat pushed back as far as
it would go.

The next 10 days of waiting were hard. But I was disci-
plined, and didn't do a home pregnancy test. I took the blood
test at the clinic at 7 a.m., then Nick and I went for breakfast
at a lovely café nearby called Patisserie Valerie. We both
ordered scrambled eggs and bacon, but I was too nervous to
eat. The call came and it was positive. I couldn't process the
enormity of it. If we hadn't pushed to have the operation, if
we hadn't kept going with treatment, we never would have
had this incredible news.

A few weeks later, we discovered that we were having twins, and Mia and Milly were born by Caesarean section at 38 weeks. It was a surprise, as we had thought we were having at least one boy, but it was an incredibly good one. We both feel so privileged to be parents, when we'd been so close to it never happening.

Q: WHAT'S YOUR ADVICE TO ANYONE DIAGNOSED WITH A LOW OR ZERO SPERM COUNT?

See a specialist and find out all the possible options. We went to our GP to discuss the first set of sperm-test results. He's a great GP, but not a fertility specialist. He just said, 'You must be devastated,' and that there was no way Nick could father his own children. I'm really pushy until I'm completely convinced; I thought: that can't be it – there must be some new technology that can help us. It was only when I asked to be referred to a urologist that we got a more detailed picture.

Q: WHAT DID YOU TELL FRIENDS ABOUT WHY YOU HAD TO HAVE IVF?

At first, we didn't tell anyone anything. Once we decided to tell a few close friends we were having treatment, after our first failure, everything became a lot easier. Before, I'd felt as if I was lying all the time. Everyone in our group was so supportive and it was amazing how many people knew people who'd been through it. We didn't tell them why we had to have IVF though – people naturally assumed the problem was on my side, and we let them.

Q: HOW DO YOU THINK A ZERO SPERM COUNT DIAGNOSIS AFFECTED YOUR HUSBAND?

I suppose all men who want children worry, to some extent, about their fertility and whether they're going to be able to father a baby. After Nick's diagnosis, but before anyone else knew we were trying, I remember a guy at a wedding telling us his wife was pregnant, joking he had 'ace swimmers'. Even though it was in jest, it hurt. Nick is very down to earth and practical, so he doesn't talk very much about his emotions, but I know he found it hard to take. His reaction was to shut down and not want to talk. I didn't push him: I read some good advice that said men can talk about fertility for a maximum of three days, and then they want to move on. I'm lucky because, when I needed to talk, I could go to my mum, sister and friends.

Q: WHAT WOULD YOU HAVE DONE IF YOU HADN'T GOT PREGNANT?

The idea of sperm donation seemed very alien to me, whereas adoption seemed more natural. At the time, I also thought it would be easier, though I've since found out it can take a lot longer.

Q: WHAT'S YOUR BEST ADVICE FOR ANYONE HAVING IVF?

Make sure you rest properly after embryo transfer. Your body has been through a lot, and so have you. And you want to give yourself the best chance. For the first week after the third transfer, I went to stay with my mum. Not that Nick didn't look after me, but I knew that if I was at home, I'd end up doing housework. Mum made me lie down and did everything for me.

The other piece of advice is, don't test early, as you can get the wrong result. I met a girl at the clinic who'd done a home test that showed up positive, but her blood test showed very low levels of pregnancy hormones, and it turned out to be a negative in the end.

● ● ● ● ● ● ● ● ●

Looking for people to speak to for the book, I tried to find a man to interview whose child had been conceived using donor sperm and whose partner had had IVF. Even though there are thousands of children conceived using donor sperm every year, I couldn't find one. Perhaps ICSI has meant a drop in the numbers of male–female couples using donor sperm. Or perhaps men just don't want to talk. It's interesting that of the couples I spoke to whose infertility was partly or wholly 'male factor', all of them allowed friends and family to think that the issue was the woman's.

Fertility coach, Anya Sizer, says she always recommends the website mensfe.net, which is dedicated to male fertility issues, as a good source of information and support. It appears (as a generalisation) that men prefer not to share in the same way that women do on fertility websites; there are a lot fewer posts on the forums, but each one has been viewed hundreds, sometimes thousands, of times. Mensfe.net is an excellent website and includes personal stories, as well as information on vasectomy reversal, sperm donation and nutrition, plus questions answered by doctors and a section on the emotional effects of fertility problems.

As regards nutrition, the latest research shows that it may be worth men whose partners are having fertility treatment taking antioxidant supplements, such as vitamin E, L-carnitine, zinc and magnesium, although it's not proven which particular supplements are most effective. That's the conclusion of a 2011 Cochrane Review of 34 randomised controlled trials involving 2876 couples.[4]

The Donor Conception Network (donor-conception-network.org) has a section aimed at men that includes personal stories. If you've been told that your best option is donor insemination, it's recommended you have counselling first. And be clear about your legal situation: in law, if you are married, you (the 'intended' father) are automatically the legal father if your child has been conceived by donated sperm, but that's not always the case if you're unmarried. (See www.nataliegambleassociates.com for more information.)

Infertility Network UK have a very useful factsheet on exactly how ICSI works, one on male infertility generally and one on the emotional side of male infertility (www.infertilitynetworkuk.com). For a full-length account of IVF from a male point of view, read *Test Tubes and Testosterone: A Man's Journey Into Infertility and IVF* by Michael Saunders (Nell James Publishers). 'The idea behind my story was just to get men talking about fertility. I imagine it will be bought by women and hopefully read by men,' says Saunders.

I had premature ovarian failure

• • • • • • • • • • •

What happens when you start trying for a baby, then find out that you are having an early menopause and that your hope of any fertility treatment working has just plummeted?

The accepted statistic is that one in 100 women has her menopause by the age of 40 (usually called premature ovarian failure, or POF). However, a new study from Imperial College, London, puts the number much higher, closer to one in 14, including those who have had surgery or treatment for cancer.[5] POF can be devastating, even for women who've finished their families. A friend I interviewed, who had her menopause at 37, said, 'Not only was I having hot flushes, feeling angry and putting on weight, but I was doing it ten or fifteen years before my friends, so there was no one to talk to about it. It didn't seem fair.'

Although, when you think of the menopause, you probably think of the typical symptoms my friend described, what it actually means for a woman is that she has gone through her store of eggs. 'At birth, your lifetime supply of eggs – your ovarian reserve – is already determined,' says Professor Bill Ledger, Professor of Obstetrics and Gynaecology at the University of Sheffield. You release one egg every 90 seconds – one of which matures each month – and when your store is gone, it's gone. 'Ovarian reserve can be reduced by ovarian cysts, surgery on an ovary, chemotherapy and radiotherapy. You also speed up the rate it reduces by drinking too much and smoking,' says Professor Ledger. But, for half of all women who have POF, no reason is usually found. 'My guess is that women who have an early menopause probably have a smaller lifetime supply of eggs to start with,' he says.

An early menopause often runs in families – so if it's happened to your mother and grandmother, it's more likely to happen to you too. Early menopause wasn't such an issue for our grannies, of course, who tended to have their children younger, but the average age of new motherhood in the UK is now almost 30. 'Mum had her babies in her 20s,' says Toni, whose story is below, 'so even if she had had an early menopause, it wouldn't have made any difference to the number of babies she could have. I thought I had at least another five years until I needed to worry.'

If you are showing signs of being peri-menopausal (you aren't actually classified as menopausal until you haven't had a period for a year), the first test your GP will usually do is for FSH (follicle-stimulating hormone), a hormone produced by the pituitary gland at the base of your brain. As the supply of eggs dwindles, this goes up. A result of 10 and under is usually considered fertile. 'But it's a very imprecise tool for looking at ovarian reserve,' says Professor Ledger. 'By the time FSH has reached over twelve, in many cases ovarian reserve has gone down very substantially.'

Two more accurate ways of measuring ovarian reserve are the antral follicle scan, which counts the number of potential follicles in your ovaries each month, and a blood test for AMH (anti-Müllerian hormone), a hormone that's directly released by the follicles in the ovary. Even if your AMH is low, it doesn't mean IVF won't work. 'But it is a warning sign you may not have a good response,' says Professor Ledger.

• • • • • • • • •

Toni, a sales manager from Manchester, had just married David when she was told, aged 31, that she was close to the end of her fertility.

Two weeks after David and I got back from honeymoon, I called my mum, to say that my period was two days late. David and I had agreed to try for babies at some point in the next few years, but I was surprised it had happened without us trying. 'Well, I'd rather be pregnant now than find out in two years that we can't have children,' I said, and we laughed. But my period came a couple of days later.

Before the wedding, my periods had been very regular and I'd never even had PMT. Then, I started to feel really down, which isn't at all like me. And I was having hot flushes, too. When I mentioned it to friends, they said I was probably having post-wedding blues, a comedown after the big event.

I went to see my GP, and mentioned, jokingly, that it might be the menopause. I was only 31, after all. He did some blood tests and rang me the next week while I was driving to work. I put him on speakerphone and heard him say, bluntly, 'Actually, it is the menopause.' He told me that my FSH was 68, when it should be 10 or below. Then he said, 'In fact, that level is post-menopausal.'

It was such a huge shock. I remember it was pouring with rain, the windscreen wipers were going, and I couldn't seem to see to process the news. At home, David comforted me, and promised me everything would be fine. But I couldn't even look at myself in the mirror because I'd think: that's a menopausal woman. How can I look so normal, when I'm not?

My GP referred me to hospital for more blood tests and scans. The results confirmed what he'd told me: menopause. The fertility specialist told me there was nothing they could do. She said we could try IVF, but we probably wouldn't succeed as my problem was going to be getting eggs. And there was no way I had two years of fertility left to wait on the NHS list. She suggested the Lister Fertility Clinic in London, as they specialise in IVF for women with menopausal hormone levels. 'But if you want to get pregnant really your only option is egg donation,' she said, 'so I suggest you have counselling for that.'

That was too hard to accept, that our only way to have a baby would be with someone else's eggs. I knew David was upset, scared that we'd never have children too. But he didn't show it; he just tried to be strong for me, because I was so completely devastated. The fact my body didn't work was all I could think about. I felt half a person and guilty – as if I'd let David down, and I wasn't the woman he married.

I fantasised about running away from everyone, emigrating to the other side of the world, alone. But the sensible me thought, I want David to have a child, and I want my parents to be grandparents. I had told Mum and some of my closest friends my diagnosis, and they were brilliantly supportive. Between them and David, I managed to keep going.

It was taking months to get appointments on the NHS so I went to see a private gynaecologist, who did more blood tests. For a change, a nice surprise: my FSH had gone down to 10. So I wasn't totally menopausal. In fact, over the next year, my FSH fluctuated between 2 and 60. It wasn't all good news, as my oestrogen was high when my FSH was low, another menopausal sign. But, the gynaecologist said, the official definition of the menopause is a year without a period, and I was still having some periods, which meant I was still ovulating, if only sometimes. So, in fact, I had what's called premature ovarian failure (POF), and there was hope. 'It just means it's going to be very, very difficult for you to get pregnant and to keep the baby,' the gynaecologist said.

My next test was a scan of my ovaries, called an antral follicle count, where they look at the number of possible follicles developing that month; it's an indicator of your ovarian reserve, how many eggs you have left. My right ovary was inactive and very small. (When I was 16, I had a cyst removed from it, and I don't think it had worked since, even though doctors told me it shouldn't have made a difference.) But, amazingly, the scan showed I was about to ovulate from my left ovary.

We were delighted, and set about making a baby that night. Two weeks later, I did a test and I was pregnant. It was absolutely brilliant, a huge relief. I thought to myself: what are they all talking about? Menopause? What nonsense. Not only was I pregnant, but the pregnancy hormones overtook the menopausal ones so, for the first time in ages, I actually felt normal.

At seven weeks, I had a private scan, and saw the heartbeat. But at 10 weeks, I went for a scan at the NHS fertility clinic and, after looking for a minute or so, the woman scanning me said, quite casually, 'There's no baby'. I said, 'Oh yes there is, I know I'm pregnant, I've seen the heartbeat.' 'No,' she said, 'there's no baby.'

David wasn't with me; I'd thought this was just a routine NHS appointment. It hurt so much, I wanted to scream, 'Do you realise what this means? You're telling me my only chance of getting pregnant has ended in a miscarriage.' I put on my knickers and tights, went to the toilet, and threw up everything I'd eaten that morning.

It turned out the baby had died around seven weeks, shortly after the first scan. I was given the choice of pills or an operation to remove what was left. I went home, took the pills and waited. The bleeding was really heavy for a week, then stopped, then started again. I went to see my GP about the bleeding, and again a few weeks later, but I was told it was normal.

For two months, I bled really heavily, huge clots, every day. Eventually, because I'd become so anaemic, I passed out at my sister's house the day before Christmas Eve, and had to be rushed to A & E. It turned out a bit of the pregnancy tissue had been left behind, and it was signalling to my body that I was still pregnant. I had a D & C (dilatation and curettage – where my womb lining was scraped out, including the left-behind pregnancy tissue) under general anaesthetic.

It felt as if I'd used up my last egg and our one chance to have a baby. Every period after that was a mixed blessing: I'd think it might be my last one, but at least it meant I had ovulated again.

I booked in for an IVF consultation at the Lister. I saw Mr Hossam Abdalla, the medical director, who was realistic, but not as fatalistic as previous doctors I'd seen. He put my odds of getting pregnant at 5 per cent, with a high chance of a miscarriage. A lot of clinics won't even take on patients with POF. (The problem is that the drugs they give you during IVF to boost your egg production are, in fact, the same hormone – FSH – that your body is overproducing because of the menopause.) Mr Abdalla said that giving me extra FSH might not make me ovulate, but it would be my best chance of getting pregnant, and at least I'd be closely monitored.

So we embarked on IVF with the highest amount of drugs possible. I wasn't hopeful. I knew the odds were against me, but I was really determined. I kept thinking of older women who get pregnant, like Cherie Blair. My mantra was: 'As long as there's one egg, I can get pregnant.'

I enjoyed the whole process of IVF. I'm not a control freak, but I liked the fact that, for the first time in ages, I knew exactly what was going on. By now, my menopausal side effects – feeling exhausted, hot flushes, brain fog, being so angry I wanted to chuck things out of the window – had got so bad that I actually felt better taking the IVF drugs.

Scans showed I had three follicles growing on my left side (and I only needed one, I kept telling myself). But when it came to egg collection, only one egg was mature enough and it was damaged. So that was the end of that.

We licked our wounds, and decided to carry on. I was absolutely not going to give up. For as long as I was ovulating, we were going to try.

By then, I'd read everything I could find on fertility, gone completely teetotal, given up caffeine and switched to organic food. I'd started to have weekly reflexology and acupuncture too. I felt panicky though, as no matter what I did, my periods – and so ovulation – were beginning to get less regular. Sometimes two months would go past without any sign of one.

I carried on at the Lister, doing cycle monitoring, so we'd know the best time to have sex. But treatment wasn't cheap; we'd already spent around £7000 on IVF, £100 a week on reflexology and acupuncture, £100 a scan and more for blood tests too, and I knew we couldn't carry on spending this kind of money indefinitely.

At the time, it seemed as if all my friends were getting pregnant around me, as if I was surrounded by bumps and prams. And I had this feeling of guilt that was weighing me down all the time. I was putting on weight and every time I had a hot flush, a fit of anger or woke up at 5 a.m., it was a reminder that I was menopausal and couldn't get pregnant. My only consolation was the thought that if I didn't get pregnant, we could try egg donation or adoption. I wasn't ready to stop trying for my own biological child just yet, but not having children at all wasn't an option.

That September, six months later, we started a new cycle of IVF. I did the injections for the usual two weeks but there was no sign of a single egg this time. Another full week of injections later, there was finally one egg there. I was fully expecting that we'd have to abandon the cycle completely. And, as I'd expected, the doctor advised us that the risk of damaging our only egg by taking it out was too high. But he had an idea: he suggested that we do IUI, where David's sperm would be put inside my uterus at exactly the right moment. Great, I thought. At least we have one option. So I did the injection to make me ovulate, started on progesterone suppositories, and we had the IUI procedure two days later.

I put the fact that I had begun to feel different down to the progesterone. But two weeks later, on New Year's Eve, I decided to do a pregnancy test (it was a couple of days early, but I wanted to know if I could drink, after being teetotal all year), and it was positive. It was a brilliant New Year!

Still, in the back of my mind, I knew the pregnancy wasn't safe. David used to phone me from work every day and ask me how I was feeling, going through a checklist: still feeling sick? Yes. Still got sore boobs? Yes. After my 12-week scan showed a healthy baby, I did start to relax, though not completely. I loved being pregnant, the novelty of it and feeling special. I didn't take one second of it for granted. I hope I never complained about it. But just the slightest thing – bleeding and, later on, not feeling the baby move – sent me straight to the hospital for checks. It all went well though and, in September, Charlie was finally born: our dream come to life, a gorgeous little lad.

My periods became pretty regular after I stopped breast-feeding Charlie at six months, so I felt positive about getting pregnant again, and we started cycle monitoring again. We do know how lucky we are to have Charlie, and I don't want to sound ungrateful, but we both would have loved a brother or sister for him. If the pre-baby me had heard me saying that, I'm sure she would have told me to shut up and just appreciate what I have! But there is a sense we haven't finished our family, and I hate the thought of both of us being a burden to Charlie when we're older.

When Charlie was 14 months, I did get pregnant, but it ended in a miscarriage at 10 weeks. Now, he's four and starting school. I thought I'd get pregnant again naturally, but we haven't managed it. Things have really slowed down for me hormonally, and I have gone four months without a period. Six months ago, we tried injecting fertility drugs again to see if I could get an egg, but it didn't work.

David struggled for a couple of weeks after that, coming to terms with the fact we won't have any more children who are fully related to us and Charlie. Now, egg donation really is our only option. I'm on the list at a clinic in the UK, but I've got mixed feelings. I am most of the way to accepting that Charlie will be an only child, and to seeing the good side of that. It's not what we would have chosen, but it's definitely enough.

Q: WHAT HELPED YOU COME TO TERMS WITH YOUR DIAGNOSIS?

I didn't accept or come to terms with the diagnosis of an early menopause until very recently. Instead, I fixated on getting pregnant. One doctor told me that your ovaries can sometimes stop working temporarily, and then restart again. So that is what I chose to think. My desire to get pregnant was stronger than the horror of facing an early menopause, so I let that be my overriding emotion. I found out that Premature Ovarian Failure happens to one in a hundred women, and it was enough to know that I wasn't alone, without having to speak to anyone who was going through the same thing. I did look at support group websites for women with Premature Ovarian Failure, such as the Daisy Network, but only to see if there were any success stories. When I couldn't find any, I stopped.

Q: WHAT IS YOUR ADVICE TO ANYONE WITH PREMATURE OVARIAN FAILURE?

Get the symptoms treated. A month ago, I got a private referral to a doctor who specialises in POF. I had avoided doing anything about my menopausal symptoms as I hadn't wanted to interfere with getting pregnant. But I thought, enough is enough – it's time for HRT. My doctor prescribed me bioidentical HRT – body-identical forms of oestrogen and progesterone. He told me that, if it made any difference at all, HRT might have increased my chances of getting pregnant. In five years, no one had mentioned that. And, two months into taking the hormones, I feel a lot more human.

Q: WHAT'S YOUR VIEW ON EGG DONATION?

I'd say, don't rush into it. It's a big step and one that needs to be thought about carefully. And you've got time because it's the donor's fertility that matters, not yours.

I would definitely tell any child conceived by egg donation that he or she was a donor baby. But, after having Charlie, I can't make up my mind if it would be fair to have a child who wasn't fully related to him. Would he look like Charlie? I'm dark, but Charlie is blond and blue-eyed like David, so my own biological child looks nothing like me! I've no doubt I'd love the child, but how would that compare to my love for Charlie?

Then I think, well, David's family are all utterly gorgeous, and the child would be fully related to them. I'd be carrying the baby for nine months then, when the baby was born, nursing him or her. I'd probably be too busy to worry about whose eggs helped make the baby.

We have been offered three possible donors so far, who are egg-sharers, which means they're willing to give away half their eggs in return for most of the cost of their IVF treatment being paid for by the recipient of the eggs. But we've rejected all of them. The first two were blonde, and that was what put me off. Then I changed my criteria to dark-haired women only, and the perfect person came up: educated, brunette, in her early 30s. But David and I talked it over, and decided to say no. It feels quite final, but we haven't said never.

Q: WHAT WAS THE MOST USEFUL ADVICE YOU WERE GIVEN?

To be honest, all the doctors were quite negative, though I suppose they were only being realistic. My friends and family helped by telling me that I'd got pregnant once, and so I could do it again. Going to see a reflexologist was a great support, too. She used to remind me that I was still ovulating sometimes, that I wasn't fully menopausal.

• • • • • • • •

If you still have periods, some clinics will perform IVF with your own eggs, even if you have high FSH and/or low AMH. Your chance of success, of course, is low, but there is a chance as long as you're ovulating. The Lister Fertility Clinic in London (ivf.org.uk), for example, specialises in this category of women, and recommends that you start treatment as soon as you can after diagnosis. Create Health (also in London) treats women with reduced ovarian reserve. The medical director, Dr Geeta Nargund, believes that a lower-dose drug regime is often more successful in such women (see createhealth.org and Chapter 9).

The main UK charity for premature ovarian failure is the Daisy Network. They hold an annual conference with speeches by experts in premature menopause. Their website (www.daisynetwork.org.uk) has information on IVF using donated eggs, as well as adoption, surrogacy and being 'positively childless'. Another good source of information on donated eggs is the Donor Conception Network (donor-conception-network.org). See pages 172–3 for more information on egg donation. And make sure you tell your doctor that you're considering egg donation, as it may affect your treatment for menopausal symptoms.

The International Premature Ovarian Failure Association (ipofa.org) has a useful factsheet too. And you may want to see a counsellor or consider therapy. To find a counsellor or therapist, go to bica.net, bacp.co.uk, psychotherapy.org.uk and bps.org.uk.

I couldn't give my son a sibling

• • • • • • • • • • • •

If conceiving your first child was as simple as putting your Pill in the bin, or was even a happy accident, finding out you can't get pregnant again can be harder than you'd imagine. Fertility coach, Anya Sizer, says that women often assume they should pull themselves together when they already have one child, and that not having a second or third can be dismissed as less upsetting than having no children at all. The poor relation of primary infertility, if you like.

'I don't think there's much sympathy for women with secondary infertility,' she says. 'Maybe you're at the school gates being a mum, so people assume you should be fine. When that was me, I was very grateful for my first child, but the fact I couldn't conceive for a second time still made me feel as if I was walking around with a black cloud over my head.'

For a woman who desperately wants that second child, but can't get or stay pregnant, it can feel as if there is a huge hole in her family. 'In fact, secondary infertility can be harder to accept than primary infertility,' says Dr Lee Lim, Consultant in Obstetrics and Gynaecology, Oxford Fertility Unit. 'And families who really want a sibling for the first child are under extra pressure when they compare themselves to friends who are having their second or third baby.'

There are lots of reasons for not wanting a single-child family: maybe you didn't like being an only child yourself, or you come from a big family. Sadly, secondary infertility is as common as primary. 'Of those who had no problems getting pregnant the first time around, around 15 per cent have problems the second time,' says Dr Lim.

Of course, it's not officially infertility until you've been trying for a year, even if you got pregnant easily the first time. 'You need to give yourself a year before you label yourself as having a problem,' says Dr Lim. 'Often, people who come to see me are anxious, and I need to explain that each month, their chances of pregnancy are only 30 to 35 per cent.'

Secondary infertility is also less likely to be due to underlying physical issues than primary infertility. 'The family dynamic can change after a first baby, so you may not have intercourse so often,' says Dr Lim. 'Or you could have experienced a difficult birth, which can be a very good natural contraceptive, as childbirth is so intimately related to the birth canal. You might not realise that you're avoiding sex or why. One sign of childbirth trauma is that you may have had a problem in attaching with your baby. A gynaeocologist isn't always the best person to help you talk about this; a counsellor can be better.'

Having said that, there are often physical reasons for secondary infertility. If you have a new partner, it may be down to his sperm (although that's not strictly secondary infertility). If you're still breastfeeding, you may not be ovulating regularly. Another risk is scar tissue in the uterus, which can happen if you have an operation, post-miscarriage.

'A telltale sign is that your periods have changed after this procedure,' says Dr Lim. Or it could be that you have or have had an infection that has blocked your tubes. Secondary infertility can also be caused by problems with your previous pregnancy and delivery, including infection, as well as other problems such as endometriosis, PCOS and fibroids.

But the reason that surprises most patients, says Dr Lim, is that a woman may be less fertile because she's put on weight after having a child. 'If your body mass index [BMI – a calculation that assesses your weight, taking into account your height] is over 30, it's much harder to get pregnant.'

Weight is often an issue for women with PCOS, as weight gain is part of the syndrome. 'Even if we have been able to help a woman with PCOS ovulate the first time around using medication if, by the time she is trying for her second baby, she has put on weight, it gets much harder,' says Dr Lim.

Finally, there's the question of age. If, for example, you had your first child at 35, by the time you get round to having your second or third, your fertility will have reduced naturally. 'It's not uncommon now for women to try for their second baby at 40 and, at that age, it's always going to be more difficult to get pregnant,' says Dr Lim. And, as your fertility is uniquely personal, it could happen earlier too. Abby, who tells her story below, got pregnant easily at 33 but, just two years later, found she couldn't get pregnant again.

The investigations for secondary infertility are the same as for any infertility, and may include blood tests and scans to check hormone levels and that you're ovulating properly, an internal examination and tests to check your Fallopian tubes are still working. And your partner will need a sperm test, as both quantity and quality can decline with age.

• • • • • • • • •

It wasn't until Abby, 37, a TV producer and writer from London, started trying for a second baby that she had problems.

I didn't even have to think about whether having two children was right for John, my husband, and me. I had always envisaged lots of kids running around. It took around seven months for me to get pregnant with Jake, my first baby, when I was 33. I really threw myself into motherhood and loved it so much that I remember thinking, five months in, I really want this again. So when Jake was 14 months, we started trying for a second baby.

But, month after month, I didn't get pregnant. I started using ovulation kits and, I admit, became completely obsessed with pregnancy. It was all I wanted and it consumed my thoughts. At any given time, if you'd asked me, I could have told you exactly where I was on my cycle. The two weeks after ovulation were the worst, when I'd constantly be thinking about whether I was pregnant or not. But the signs of being pregnant are the same signs as getting your period – for me, bloating and tender breasts – so every month, it was a mental and emotional nightmare. On the day of my best friend's wedding I was due to get my period and spent the whole day wondering if I would come on or not. Of course, I did.

Whenever I got my period, I'd have an awful crash. It was as if I was properly, clinically depressed; I would go back to bed for the first and second day and cry for most of the time. I remember coming down for breakfast and sobbing and sobbing in front of John. He was understanding, but he couldn't really comprehend the heady combination of a bitter disappointment plus a hormonal crash that made me feel so low.

Sex became something that was difficult to deal with as a couple. Exactly when I ovulated began to control our sex life. Scheduled sex is like sitting down to dinner when all the food is ready, but you're not hungry. We were no longer a normal couple having normal sex, because I was always thinking about the end goal.

Like me, John wanted two children but he would have been absolutely fine to wait a year and see what happened. So why did I get into such a fertility frenzy? There were a few reasons. We seemed to be surrounded by lots of breeding people. Because my friends (in fact, my generation of women, in general) were starting their families slightly later, everyone I knew was having their babies close together, one after the other. Unable to do the same, I saw myself as desperate, and felt that other people were looking at me, pitying me, thinking: poor her, she can't conceive again.

Also, having got pregnant relatively easily before, I couldn't understand why it should be taking so long this time. Plus, not only was I thinking about pregnancy all the time, I'd met a few other mums who were having problems the second time too, so I'd begun to talk about it all the time.

Life became all about pregnancy. I was reading different advice on the internet every day, taking handfuls of various supplements, having fresh wheatgrass juice every morning and weekly reflexology and acupuncture sessions. Looking back, it had become a full-time job. I couldn't stop thinking that there must be something we weren't doing which could increase our chances.

A year after we started trying, I made an appointment at a fertility clinic for us to get checked out. John's sperm was a little bit below par, but not too bad. My tubes were clear and my FSH was under 10, but when the doctor did a scan to look at my antral follicle count, to see how many potential follicles I had that month, I only had one or two on each ovary.

He told me that my ovaries looked more like those of a woman in her mid-40s, and I was only 37. Then I had an AMH blood test, another way to measure ovarian reserve, and my level was classified as 'low' too. That took the stress up a notch. Finding out there *was* actually something wrong was very emotional. It began to look less and less likely that I'd get pregnant.

As my tubes were open, so – in theory – the sperm could travel to fertilise the egg as in a natural pregnancy, doctors told me I might not need IVF, but was a good candidate for stimulated IUI (where you do hormone injections, the same as IVF, and on the day your eggs are ripe, they insert the sperm into your womb). Injecting the drugs made me feel out of it, not quite on this planet.

Even though I was open with close friends about having treatment, I still felt very alone. And I had to carry on with life as normal, looking after Jake and the house. It was a strain, though, and I remember on one occasion having a huge argument with my mum. I complained to her that Jake was being difficult, and she said it might have been because he was picking up vibes from me. I over-reacted and got really angry, telling her she was out of order.

The first cycle, I over-responded and produced too many eggs. That meant I had to have a horrible procedure called aspiration, where they pop the follicles via a tube that goes into your womb through your cervix. I was awake the whole time, and it was grim. I don't think I'd realised what I was getting myself into with the stimulated IUI cycles. It was much more medical and full on than I'd expected.

What was amazing though, is how John and I totally came together once we'd started treatment. It became one of the best times of our relationship. He kept telling me it was the right thing to do, and I felt really supported. John never questioned any of the bills either. We were spending so much money, it didn't seem real – £700 one day, £500 the next. What struck me about fertility treatment is that if it doesn't work, it feels like a complete waste of money. If it does work, it's money very well spent. After all, I'd rather have a baby than a new kitchen.

After three IUIs in four months, I started pushing the doctors to recommend IVF because the success rates are so much better than IUI. People say having IUI prepares you for IVF and I think it does; I had got used to the side effects of the drugs, and all the intrusive and personal medical procedures.

The lead-up to IVF was quite an ordeal, even before I started the drugs. I had to have a hysteroscopy; my doctor told me that it's not certain why, but having this procedure can help to improve the chance of implantation. The doctor also did a dummy run to check my cervix was going to be open enough for transfer by inserting a tube into it and leaving it in for a few hours.

Having found the IUIs so traumatic, when it came to IVF I really tried to prepare for it, to get revved up mentally and physically. I was scared (mainly, that it wouldn't work), but I tried to put a lot of positive energy into every procedure. I'd read a lot about whether the mind can make a difference to fertility. Even though I didn't wholly believe it, I thought, there's no harm in being positive. But I was up or down with every piece of good or bad news. Every day was a rollercoaster on IVF, not only because it's so important to get right, but because the drugs were making me spaced out too.

John was more positive. He saw IVF as a solution and he wasn't scared of it. Although he thought it might take more than one go, he also believed there was no reason why the clinic couldn't help us. He was determined to persist with treatment until we got what we wanted.

At my first scan, they only saw six follicles developing, and the doctor in charge of me said that ideally they'd like to see more. He said I was a 'slow responder', explaining that it was as though my ovaries were deaf, and needed more drugs to 'hear' the message. This was a real blow. The doctor immediately maximised my drug dosage, but not only was I disheartened, I was now terrified it wouldn't work. Afterwards, I spoke to a friend of mine who'd done IVF and had got pregnant, and she'd only had three eggs harvested; that made me feel better, and three eggs became my benchmark.

Every day, I did what the doctors said without questioning it. It's quite invasive and personal, to give someone else the task of getting you pregnant, and it all felt quite mechanical – like being on a conveyor belt – but I trusted that the doctors were doing the best they could for us.

On the day that snow brought the whole of London to a standstill, and a friend had her operation for a brain aneurysm cancelled, the fertility clinic was open, having picked up key staff around London with a helicopter.

I forced myself to view the side effects of the drugs – fuzzy thinking, tiredness – as positive, proof that something was happening. I had some bloating and my ovaries felt strange, but I told myself it was all good. By the second or third scan, things weren't looking quite so dire, as I'd gone up to eight follicles. Having the egg-collection operation was quite surreal, especially being with all the other women in the ward before and afterwards. It was odd to be sharing such a crucial moment in our lives with strangers. But it was also quite exciting. We all wished each other good luck.

When I came round from the anaesthetic, the doctor told us that every single follicle had yielded an egg – that meant we had eight, which was amazing. From then on, it became like a dream IVF cycle. Every day, the embryologist would telephone me and say positive things about the embryos. In the end, every single one of them lasted five days and went to blastocyst.

Before transfer, there was some debate about whether we should have one or two embryos put back. The embryologist was pushing for one, as the embryos were such good quality, but the doctor said we could have two. Faced with that decision in a more rational state, I'd have gone for one; as John pointed out, we already had one child, and having twins wouldn't have been practical. But at the time, I'd got myself into such a state about not being able to have a baby that I was completely up for a multiple pregnancy. I didn't even consider the medical issues for me or any babies, such as that a twin pregnancy has a higher risk of miscarriage and complications. I just desperately wanted a child or even children.

In the end, I did have two embryos put back in. One was top grade, and the other was almost as good. Transfer was horrible: I got really cold because they told me to drink what felt like gallons of water, there was no heating on and I was only wearing a flimsy gown. John did his best to keep me calm and warm.

People say the two-week wait is the hardest part, and it is. Suddenly, from doing injections, having scans, taking phone calls, you're on your own and there's no contact with the clinic. For the first three days, I stayed in bed while Jake was at nursery. One day, I'd think I was feeling pregnancy symptoms, then the next day, I wouldn't. It was like all those months when I'd hoped I was pregnant, but much more loaded.

The night before the pregnancy test, I couldn't sleep. I got up at 6 a.m. and did it in the bathroom. It was positive. I couldn't quite take it in. I went in and got into bed with John and woke him up and we hugged. It wasn't until I went into the clinic later that day that it really sank in.

I went to the six-week scan convinced it was twins. But there was only one heartbeat. It was a shock – I'd thought it would be all or nothing. The staff at the clinic and John were really delighted, but I kept thinking: what happened to the other one? It's strange, as I had a sense of loss, and even though I know it's better to have one baby at a time, I still think about the other possible baby to this day, whenever I look at beautiful Edie, who's now six months old.

The embryos turned out to be such good quality that we've got six blastocyst embryos on ice. I'm very grateful to have Jake and Edie, but I don't know if I'm up for having a third child yet – or ever. We haven't decided what we'll do with the embryos; maybe we'll donate them to medical research.

Q: HAD YOU HEARD OF SECONDARY INFERTILITY BEFORE IT HAPPENED TO YOU?

I knew some people struggled with miscarriage, but I assumed that if you'd had one child and wanted a second within a couple of years, you'd be fine. I didn't really listen to talk about declining fertility; I thought it alarmist when I heard doctors saying that after the age of 35 your fertility 'falls off a cliff'. Certainly, I will tell my children what happened to me, so they can make up their minds about when to try for their own family.

Q: WHAT'S YOUR ADVICE TO SOMEONE WHO'S STRUGGLING TO CONCEIVE AFTER HAVING A CHILD?

People say, 'Oh, you have a child, you should be grateful.' And yes, you are so grateful, but you are also devastated to think that might be it. It's important to acknowledge what you're going through; I think the frustration and disappointment must be every bit as acute as not being able to conceive the first time. If you already have a child, you know what you're missing. And your idea of a family is being torn to shreds.

You have to keep plugging away with trying, giving yourself breaks from treatment when you need to, as it's very intense. Most importantly, keep the faith. My husband helped me with this. And now we have a daughter, we are just so delighted and grateful, with her, for ourselves and for Jake. IVF made the experience of her so much more special – a reward for all our hard work.

Q: WHAT'S YOUR ADVICE TO SOMEONE WHO'S CONSIDERING HAVING IVF FOR SECONDARY INFERTILITY?

Don't be scared of it. It's perceived in society as a much bigger deal than it really is. When you've got to the point that you need IVF, you've done a lot of the hard work by having all the fertility tests and maybe IUI. You've already been sad and had to deal with a lot of uncertainty. Before I had IVF, I had the attitude that it was high-tech and unnatural, but it's really not that bad. The best way to think about it is simply that IVF gives you a better chance.

Q: WHAT PRACTICAL THINGS HELPED YOU TO GET THROUGH IVF?

Much as I hated having the IUI cycles before IVF, they gave me an opportunity to learn what not to do during IVF. I tried to live as normal a life as possible during IUI – for example, I was in the pub all afternoon on my birthday, when I should have been resting. But when it came to IVF, I focused on it completely and didn't let anything get in the way.

Also, at first I tried every complementary therapy going, but, by the time I got to doing IVF, I knew what was working for me – acupuncture. I tried to be really healthy but not

obsessed, so, very occasionally, I'd have a small glass of wine.
I also tried to stay calm.

Q: IS IT A GOOD THING TO TALK TO FRIENDS ABOUT WHAT YOU'RE GOING THROUGH?

I found it was a release to let people know what we were
doing. That said, at some points it's better to get on with
things yourself and not talk about them so much. Sometimes,
with other women who are also trying to get pregnant, it can
become destructive, as you end up comparing yourself to
them. I had one friend who I confided in, who was going
through the same thing, and who was incredibly supportive.

• • • • • • • • •

There's not nearly so much written about secondary infertility as primary. Fertilityzone.co.uk have a dedicated secondary infertility section on their forum and reading the posts
shows how difficult it can be. One mum says, 'I am so glad to
have my son, he is my life and I wouldn't want to be without
him, but I can't get rid of this agonising pain in my heart. I
want another baby … I so desperately want my son to have a
sibling.' Fertility Friends (fertilityfriends.co.uk) also has a
very busy thread on their forum for secondary infertility.

In their explanation of secondary infertility, the National
Infertility Association in the US, Resolve (resolve.org),
describe all the aspects in a very perceptive way: 'It's a cruel
irony that the more positively parents feel about parenting,
the more painful is their experience of secondary infertility'
(www.resolve.org/diagnosis-management/infertility-
diagnosis/secondary-infertility.html). They also bring up the
issue of how wanting another child and having treatment can
affect the child you already have.

Lynda, 42, blogs at http://tryingfornumbertwo.blogspot. com/ about almost five years spent trying for a sibling for her daughter, who she conceived after only three months. She is appealingly honest: 'It seems so unfair that for most of my daughter's life I have been grieving for an unborn child. I really feel that my grief has overshadowed the joy of having my beautiful daughter.' Kathy Benson, now mother to Sean and Abby, went through four years of secondary infertility and documents her journey in her blog, chicagobenson. blogspot.com. 'I especially had a hard time', she writes, 'when friends and family members would announce their pregnancies publicly at social gatherings.' She also makes the point that women with secondary infertility tend to be surrounded by reminders that they can't conceive because they are so often around children and other mothers. The book she found most useful was *Conquering Infertility: Dr. Alice Domar's Mind/Body Guide to Enhancing Fertility and Coping With Infertility* (Penguin Books).

On the practical side, Infertility Network UK has a factsheet on secondary infertility, available at infertilitynetworkuk.com. Sadly, if you already have a child, it's very unlikely that fertility treatment such as IVF or ICSI will be NHS-funded.

Cancer affected
my fertility

· · · · · · · · · · · ·

I t seems particularly unfair that if someone has endured
the uncertainties of cancer and the difficulties of treatment, that she or he could also end up infertile too, as a
result. Sometimes the cancer itself is to blame, but more
usually it's down to surgery, radiotherapy and/or
chemotherapy.

Fertility preservation is now usually offered before cancer
treatment. For men, sperm can be frozen and stored before
treatment, then used in IVF, usually ICSI. If sperm wasn't
stored – for example, if the man had cancer in childhood –
then he may be able to have sperm extracted from his testes
during an operation, frozen, then the couple can have ICSI
later on (see Chapter 2).

The most tried-and-tested fertility preservation technique
for women is to have IVF prior to cancer treatment, and the
embryos frozen, to use when you're better. 'Of course, this is
not always possible if the patient doesn't have a partner,' says
Mr Tarek El-Toukhy, Consultant and Honorary Lecturer in

Reproductive Medicine and Surgery at Guy's and St Thomas' Hospital NHS Foundation Trust. If that's the case, she may have the option of freezing her eggs, though this is less established and, until a few years ago, fewer eggs than embryos survived the freezing and thawing process. A new freezing technique called vitrification has boosted the thaw rate of eggs; recently, the first two British babies were born from eggs frozen using this technique, at the Midland Fertility Services clinic.

If the cancer has a hormonal element, as some kinds of breast and ovarian cancer do, or the cancer needs immediate treatment, IVF beforehand might not be possible. 'In some cancers, it's not safe to have ovarian stimulation,' says Mr El-Toukhy. 'There are other options we can offer, including preserving ovarian tissue by freezing it. But at this stage it is experimental, and very few babies have been born from it worldwide.' The idea of this treatment is that the ovarian tissue can be put back inside the woman's body to grow eggs when she's well, or in future, the immature eggs inside the tissue might even be matured in a test tube and used in IVF.

Of course, there is no guarantee that any assisted reproduction technique will work. 'The clinician has to talk to the patient openly about what treatments they can offer, and the realistic chance of achieving a pregnancy,' says Mr El-Toukhy. 'But you could argue that a chance is better than no chance.'

Some women do still have functioning ovaries after treatment for cancer, which means they can have IVF if needed, or even get pregnant naturally. 'There are a lot of factors that affect whether the patient retains her ovarian function – the type of cancer, the age of the patient and her ovarian reserve, whether she had surgery, radiotherapy and chemotherapy, the type of chemotherapy, the number of courses of chemotherapy and, of course, how badly the cancer has affected her general health,' says Mr El-Toukhy. If cancer does affect fertility, there may be the option of egg donation or surrogacy.

Sadly, although IVF and embryo freezing are routinely provided on the NHS, the rest of these treatments often need to be paid for.

• • • • • • • • •

Lucy, 32, a hospital manager from Hampshire, thought she might never have her own child after cancer.

My husband John and I came out of the hospital, got straight into a cab and went to have a slap-up celebration lunch in Gordon Ramsay's restaurant in Chelsea. We had good reason to celebrate: we'd just been told that we could go ahead with IVF and surrogacy. Just 10 months earlier, I'd been diagnosed with a rare form of cancer in my womb. I hadn't even been sure if I'd still be around, and hadn't dreamed I'd be fertile.

It had all started two years before, when John and I had been delighted to find out that I was pregnant. But I had the worst morning sickness, constant vomiting and no energy. I couldn't eat or drink anything without throwing it up. I felt hungover, but multiplied by a million.

When I went for a scan at 10 weeks, the sonographer could see immediately that there was something wrong. In place of the expected embryo, there were a lot of fluid-filled cysts, like a little bunch of grapes. The doctor came in and said, 'I'm sorry, but there's no baby.' He told me I had a molar pregnancy, where the fertilisation of an egg goes wrong, and it turns into a mass of cells that grow very rapidly, but don't form the foetus and placenta of a normal pregnancy. It would need to be surgically removed. He added that there was a 10 per cent chance that the cells would continue to grow after surgery – a rare form of pregnancy-related cancer.

We were so hung up on there being no baby that we couldn't take in the cancer part at first. Later on, a more senior doctor explained it to us again, and two days later, I had an operation to remove the molar pregnancy. Though I was upset about losing the pregnancy, I was relieved when the surgery was over.

But, two weeks later, I started getting really strong abdominal pains, and I was admitted to hospital and prescribed morphine. The next day, I was transferred to Charing Cross Hospital, the national screening centre for molar pregnancy, where I had every kind of chest X-ray and chest and abdominal CT scan.

The first thing the consultant there said to me was that I had cancer. Molar pregnancies produce incredibly high levels of beta hCG, the pregnancy hormone (that explained my awful morning sickness). After having the molar pregnancy removed, my level should have gone down to zero, but lab tests showed it was still close to a million (in a healthy pregnancy, it wouldn't normally go above 280,000). I was one of the unlucky 10 per cent whose molar pregnancy had turned into a form of cancer.

On the ward, away from home, I felt lonely and scared. And I was still in pain. But the doctors were upbeat about my chances: they told me that chemotherapy had a 99 per cent success rate.

I started having chemotherapy every two weeks – injections of a drug called methotrexate that would kill the remaining abnormal placental tissue. It took five months for the chemotherapy to work, for my hCG levels to get back to normal. The side effects weren't too bad: my eyes were sore and I felt a bit tired and run down, but it was bearable.

I was told not to get pregnant for a year, as the hCG produced by the pregnancy would interfere with my monitoring. That was hugely frustrating, as John and I wanted to get on with life. I went back to work as a hospital manager and we decided to make the most of the year: I went on a spending spree: I bought a brand new Mazda MX5, spent a fortune on manicures, pedicures, fake tans, massages, handbags, designer shades, ate out at some swanky London restaurants and went to the theatre, the British Grand Prix and to see Chelsea, John's favourite team. We also booked a holiday to the Maldives – something else to look forward to.

But we never got to go.

My abdominal pain came back and I ended up having three operations to treat it that year. First, the surgeon performed a laparoscopy and found that the inside of my abdomen was filled with adhesions (pelvic adhesions are bands of tissue that stick tissue and organs together – a kind of internal scar tissue that can be caused by an operation, among other things). The second time, he had to open me up completely to get rid of the adhesions. That's when he saw that my left Fallopian tube had come away from my uterus and had got caught up in my bowel. The left ovary had also died because its blood supply had been cut off, so he had to remove it.

I was terrified that with only one ovary, my chances of conceiving would be halved, but the doctors explained that it wouldn't alter my chances, as the Fallopian tube next to my remaining ovary was clear.

I tried to move on, but just a few months later, the pain came back. In my next operation, the surgeon removed a blood clot from under my right Fallopian tube.

Just a week after the operation, on my 30th birthday, we had an amazing weekend, cocktails and dinner at Claridges. We stayed over in a beautiful room, with a massive marble bathroom and one of those showers where you feel as though you're standing in the heaviest rain. It was really special. Both John and I thought that I was finally better.

Then, a month later, in the run-up to Christmas, I suspected I might be pregnant. I did a home test and it was positive. It was great news, but I was also freaked out and kept saying, 'I don't want to get sick again'. I didn't feel nearly as nauseous as when I'd had the molar pregnancy, which was a good sign, I thought. But, driving on the motorway in the New Year, I felt the most unbearable sharp pain in my abdomen, and thought I was going to pass out.

I turned back and drove straight to my GP who suspected it might be an ectopic pregnancy (where the foetus develops in a Fallopian tube), so I was admitted to our local hospital. They monitored my hCG level, to see if it was going up or down. If it was going down, it was likely to be a miscarriage; if it was going up, it was likely to be an ectopic pregnancy. But it stayed exactly the same – a sign that the pregnancy wasn't viable, but also, possibly, that I might be ill again.

I was sent back up to Charing Cross. After lots more scans and tests, doctors told me they suspected I had a much more serious form of cancer. I had yet another operation – keyhole surgery to get a biopsy of the mass they had seen in my uterus on the MRI and CT scans. But what the surgeon saw with the camera didn't tally with the scans, so he decided to open me up completely, cutting up my womb to remove the mass. And thank goodness he did – 10 days later, we got the diagnosis that I had a cancer called placental site trophoblastic tumour (PSTT), but such a rare type that nobody at Charing Cross had ever seen it before.

Because the cancer was so rare, the doctors couldn't give me a prognosis. Also, the MRI scans had shown abnormalities on my spleen and remaining ovary, and until I'd had the associated lymph nodes taken out and analysed, we wouldn't know if the cancer had spread. I said to the consultant: 'Just do what you need to do, but please tell me I'm going to be ok.' And he said, 'Unfortunately, nobody knows what the future holds.' Which was when I realised how ill I was.

Treatment for the cancer would be the biggest operation of all – this time a hysterectomy, including removal of my pelvic lymph nodes and my appendix, followed by eight weeks of heavy-duty chemotherapy. We were told that the chemotherapy would very likely stop my remaining ovary from working properly and that I'd probably go into menopause.

My consultant suggested that, during the hysterectomy, a slice of my ovary could be removed and frozen. He explained that although it was experimental technology, the ovarian tissue could be used to help me produce my own eggs later on.

Having a hysterectomy at 30 is pretty horrendous, as is the thought of an early menopause, but they were minor details considering what I was facing. I was consumed by a horrible fear that I might not survive. At this point, my focus was on getting myself fit and well, and anything else – including having children – slipped into the background. What kept me going was that I had no other option – I knew I had to have the surgery and chemotherapy if I was ever to be well again.

Sitting in the hospital bed after the operation, I thought, I'll just have to get myself better now, get my ovary working and prove the doctors wrong. But I was very ill, and looked so awful that I couldn't even bear for my parents or friends to come and see me. There was some good news though: analysis of my lymph nodes showed that the cancer hadn't spread.

I can't find the words to describe how amazing John was throughout the time I was ill. While I was in Charing Cross, he gave up work for six weeks, and was with me every day. A few months before my diagnosis, determined to be well, I'd signed up for the London marathon, and because John hadn't wanted me to train on my own, he'd got a place too. While I was ill, he kept running; he said it was the best way to clear his mind.

Ten days after the operation, I started my cocktail of chemotherapy. The previous chemo was nothing compared to this. One chemo drug combination was given weekly intravenously, and for days afterwards I'd feel unbelievably exhausted. My bones ached, my stomach was upset and I'd long for the days to pass. The other had to be given overnight in hospital, and would knock me out. The first time, I woke up in the early hours of the morning feeling terrible, as if I was being melted from the inside. I begged the medical team to stop the treatment; I cried and cried until I could bear for them to continue again.

Once, the chemotherapy leaked from the drip on to my arm and burned my skin, so a plastic surgeon had to cut my arm open and flush through the burned tissue with saline to prevent any permanent tissue damage. With the cuts bandaged, it looked as if I'd slit my wrist.

As I couldn't use my hands, John even washed my hair for me. That was until my hair started to fall out. That made me feel so unfeminine, and reminded me of my illness every time I looked in the mirror. When I had to shave my head, because it looked so patchy and horrible, John shaved his in support. We looked like a pair of hooligans – like the Mitchell brothers from *EastEnders*!

One of the hardest things for me was for friends and family to know how poorly I was. It was difficult knowing that they'd be sad for me. So I kept it all to myself, even though John said I should talk about how I was feeling more.

On the days when I felt well enough to go out, John would take me to see friends or we'd pop to the pub. For a few months, I didn't feel strong or well enough to go anywhere without him. There was a point, he told me afterwards, when he worried that he'd always be my carer – and that's not what you want at 30.

After the chemotherapy, my scans and blood tests showed no sign of the cancer. As far as the doctors were concerned, my treatment was over, though I'd still need regular check-ups, and wouldn't get the final all-clear for five years.

It was just a few months later, at one of my check-ups, that we discovered my ovary had started working again, against all odds, and that my ovarian function was absolutely normal for my age, 31. So you can understand why John and I celebrated!

I was nervous about the idea of IVF, being pumped full of hormones; and the doctors all said that I'd have to do at least three cycles to expect a result. They told us to wait six months, until my body was ready and, I assume, until I was mentally strong enough too.

We booked to go to a conference on surrogacy, to find out more about it. But on the morning of the conference, John's sister, Sally, texted me to ask what we were up to that weekend, and I told her. That was the first time I'd ever let anybody (apart from my parents) know that surrogacy might be an option. She texted back, saying, 'You know you don't need to go because I'd love to help you.' Sally explained that she'd been thinking about offering earlier, but didn't want to bring it up as I'd been so private. She had finished her own family – two gorgeous boys aged eight and nine – and seeing me with them, she knew how much I loved kids, and could tell how sad we were, and how desperate to have a family.

One night a few weeks later, Sally came over, and I told her everything that had happened. We cried together and discussed how she'd feel if the baby was a girl or if there was something wrong with it. She assured me that she would consider herself simply as the oven, cooking our baby for us.

Before we could have IVF, John had to have his sperm frozen for six months as, in the eyes of the law, he'd be a sperm donor. Then, finally, I could start IVF. I couldn't face another general anaesthetic, so I asked to be awake for egg collection. Although I was sedated, it was very painful. The doctor took out three eggs. All three fertilised, but by the transfer day, only two embryos were of good enough quality to use. Sally said, 'We're only going to do this once, so put them both in.' We were disappointed that we had none to freeze, but hopeful.

When Sally called on the morning of the pregnancy test, to say it was positive, I was so excited that I ran around the hall screaming. I had to force myself to calm down, to remember it was still early days.

Sally had a lot of nausea, which she hadn't had in her two previous pregnancies, and I worried it might be a molar pregnancy. It was hard enough letting someone else carry the baby, let alone worrying that I might have made her ill too. The clinic reassured me that they only transfer normal-looking, healthy embryos, but it wasn't until the three of us went to the first scan, at nine weeks, and we saw a heartbeat, that I relaxed.

All through the pregnancy Sally made sure we were involved in all the scans and appointments. Later on, the only thing I couldn't bear to do was to feel the baby kick. A kick was too much of a wrench, a reminder that the baby should have been inside me.

I'd assumed I'd be able to take the baby home straight after the birth, but the hospital said that wouldn't be possible because the birth mother, Sally, would, at that point, be the legal mother. So the baby would have to stay with her in hospital until they were both discharged. But, they said, I wouldn't be able to stay in hospital too.

As we couldn't become the legal parents until we got a parental order – which we couldn't even apply for until six weeks after the birth – we were stuck. I asked, 'So who's going to look after the baby, because Sally certainly doesn't want to.' Sally backed me up, and that's when we spoke to Natalie Gamble, a solicitor who specialises in fertility. Legally, the hospital's decision was right, but Natalie said there was usually a pragmatic way to sort these things out without breaking the law. After some negotiation, it was agreed that I could pay for a room in the hospital for me and the baby until Sally and the baby were discharged. After that, the hospital would no longer have any say and I'd be able to take the baby home.

I was incredibly anxious leading up to the birth. How would we all feel once the long-awaited baby finally arrived? How would Sally feel when the baby came to us? How would the baby respond to us, having been inside Sally for nine months? And how would we thank Sally for giving us the most amazing gift anyone could possibly give?

As it turned out, the day was one I will treasure for ever. The baby was born by C-section, as Sally had wanted. Straight away, the nurse came over and gave her to me. It was such an amazing moment. Neither John nor I minded if she was a boy or a girl, as long as everyone was well. But seeing her beautiful little face just made me melt with joy that we had a precious little girl.

The first thing Sally said was that she was beautiful, then she told me to take Ellie to see her daddy, who was waiting outside. What could I say to that? Thank you didn't even come close.

We had to stay in hospital until Sally was discharged. Ellie and I had a private room at the opposite end of the ward to her. The next day, Sally knocked on the door and asked if she could have a cuddle with her niece, which was lovely.

Those first three days in hospital, I couldn't take my eyes off Ellie. I know I'm biased, but she *is* beautiful. It was wonderful just to sit there, holding her, and to be a mum. I hadn't wanted to stay in hospital, but it was good for us to have that quiet time together, just Ellie and me, to get to know each other.

To become Ellie's legal parents, we had to apply to the court for the parental order. An official came to our house to talk to us about how she was conceived, how we felt, if the family had accepted her. One of the things we told her was that our friends and family were amazing at welcoming Ellie into the world. Everyone loved her just as if she'd grown inside me.

I do think it must be hard for Sally. Even though she's an auntie to Ellie, she's kept in the background for the nine months since she was born. Maybe she doesn't want to be seen to be getting too close. I think it must be emotional for her, but we haven't spoken about it. We gave her a massive bunch of beautiful flowers, with a note from Ellie saying, 'Thank you for looking after me for nine months'. 'Thank you' doesn't seem good enough, but what else is there to say?

I can't remember what life was like before Ellie. Even the sleepless nights haven't bothered me. It's such a joy to see her growing into a wonderful little person. John adores her too and her little face lights up when he walks in from work.

I don't dwell on the cancer, or the fact I had to have a hysterectomy. I have a big scar, which runs from hip to hip, but it doesn't upset me. Of course, I would rather have carried my daughter myself, but I have tried to keep that in perspective. We're going to tell Ellie how she was conceived, as soon as she can understand it. We want her to know how special she is, and if she chooses to tell people in the future, that's up to her.

We have actually started thinking about another baby, although we know that Sally wouldn't be our surrogate, as it took her a while to recover from the C-section. I do wonder if we're being selfish, asking for another child, as if a surrogate chooses us, does that mean another couple would lose out? We'd need to have tests too, to make sure my ovary is still working, and we have to consider the financial implications, as Ellie cost us around £11,000.

John says we'll find the money if we have to. He's more worried about the effects on my health of having more treatment. But, with what you get at the end, it's worth it.

Q: WAS HAVING A BABY VIA A SURROGATE A HARD CHOICE TO MAKE?

I'd always imagined myself having three, four or even five children. What drove me to work so hard in my 20s was to get set up so we could have a family. Before cancer, I would never have imagined choosing to have a baby through surrogacy. But I was so thrilled to be well and alive and – against all the odds – to have the chance of a baby that was biologically our own, that the fact that someone else would have to carry it was something I was prepared to accept.

I think my parents struggled with the concept of surrogacy at the start. They were concerned about my health and how we'd cope if the IVF didn't work.

Q: HOW DID CANCER AFFECT YOU?

After the hysterectomy, I went back to work. I'd always loved my job, and thought that working would make me feel normal again. I was determined not to let the cancer change my life. That mental attitude was helpful to get me through treatment but, back at work, it meant I just wore myself out.

One morning, I woke up and I couldn't stop crying. I was pushing myself, pretending that everything was as it always had been, when really I just wanted to be a mum. I took myself off to my GP, and sat in the waiting room, tears pouring down my face. The GP said I'd tried to do too much, too soon, and that it can take two years for your body to recover from cancer and chemotherapy, let alone all the surgery I'd had. I realised that I needed to concentrate on having a family, not work, so I resigned. When I went back to see one of the specialists who'd treated me, he said, 'Once you've had cancer, your life is never the same, no matter how much you don't want it to change.' And that's so true.

Q: WHAT DID YOU TELL PEOPLE ABOUT YOUR ILLNESS?

I didn't tell my friends, apart from one, about the full extent of the surgery. I think people guessed, but I felt so embarrassed that I couldn't talk about it. Having a hysterectomy made me feel sad and inadequate because I couldn't do the one thing a woman is supposed to do. It was so hard to think that we might not be able to have children, and that made seeing friends who'd had babies difficult. I was happy for them, but it made me desperately sad to think how things had worked out for John and me. It wasn't until I knew I could have IVF that I could see them again.

Five months before the baby was due, we announced the pregnancy to our friends. They were all incredibly surprised. Not many people know anyone who's had a surrogate child, after all. I didn't go into detail about why; I just said that it was because of the cancer.

Q: WHAT WOULD YOU HAVE DONE IF YOUR OVARY HADN'T STARTED WORKING?

It would have been unbelievably painful to have had to accept that my lifelong dream of being a mum was over. I guess I'd have had to try to keep it in perspective, as I did with everything else that happened.

When we talked about our options, John said he'd be happy to use an unrelated surrogate who'd donate her egg as well as carry the pregnancy. For me, that would have been a step too far. I'd have been happier with adoption.

There is also the option of using the ovarian tissue that was removed. Although at the moment this technology is still experimental (there's one case in the UK of a woman who started to produce eggs after having the tissue re-implanted, although she didn't get pregnant) the doctors have advised us that fertility science progresses so fast that in a few years' time, using the tissue probably won't be beyond the realms of possibility.

• • • • • • • • •

Ideally, you should ask your doctor about ways to preserve your fertility before treatment. Cancerhelp.org.uk is the information site of the charity Cancer Research. Go to the 'About cancer' section, then to 'Cancer questions and answers', and select 'Sex and fertility' as the subject, and you'll find answers to a long list of common questions on fertility. Macmillan also have two information sections: one for women and one for men at Macmillan.org.uk. Plus, if you have questions, you can email via the website or call 0808 808 00 00.

Usually, only freezing embryos will be funded by the NHS, but it's worth finding out if you could appeal to your local authority (see infertilitynetworkuk.com).

At Fertilehope.org, a US site, you can use the 'options calculator' to work out the likelihood of your period stopping after cancer treatment, and the 'risk calculator' shows the effect of different treatment regimes on fertility.

Life On Ice (lifeonice.com) is a website created by Emma Leach, who was herself in the news when she had her ovarian tissue re-implanted after cancer treatment. Having previously gone into menopause, her ovary did start working again, but only for a few months. The website provides details of the most advanced forms of fertility preservation, including ovarian tissue freezing and transplantation (OTFT). 'The latest thinking is that the damage from treatment takes an average of 10 years off the fertile life of ovaries,' she says. That is, you will get the menopause 10 years early. She thinks that OTFT is the future, despite the fact that only a handful of babies have been born this way to date, and gives contact details for the few doctors worldwide who are experienced at re-implanting ovarian tissue (there are more who can operate to remove and freeze it).

I'm a single mother by choice

• • • • • • • • • • • •

A growing trend for women to make a concious decision to have a child alone means they now have their own moniker, SMC, which stands for Single Mothers by Choice. 'The figures do suggest more single women are choosing to have children on their own,' says Marilyn Crawshaw, retired Senior Lecturer in Social Work and now Honorary Fellow at the University of York. 'It's not always because time is running out, but often the woman feels that if she doesn't do something now, it will.' If that's you and IUI doesn't work, you may find yourself moving on from IUI to IVF quite quickly.

Marilyn Crawshaw thinks that by the time a woman has contacted a clinic, she has usually thought in depth about the issues of having a child alone. 'A single woman has probably been more exposed to criticism than a couple having IVF, with people saying things such as, "You're being selfish" or, "What gives you the right?" We all grow up with the message that the ideal family is the nuclear family, so going it alone can lead to some inner conflict. Counselling can be useful here for helping you explore aloud your decisions and the implications of having a baby alone without feeling judged.'

Amy, who describes how she chose to be a single mother below, says that the support of her family and friends was crucial to her decision. 'I reasoned that a lot of marriages break up in any case, so there are a lot of single mums out there not by choice. Once I'd made the decision to get pregnant, I was lucky to feel very safe in my little environment, with my family and friends.'

● ● ● ● ● ● ● ●

Amy, 42, an art consultant, knew she'd always wanted children. Finding herself single at the age of 37, she decided to go it alone.

That I wanted a baby, but my long-term partner didn't, wasn't the cause of our break-up but it was a factor. I was living in New York with a job I loved in the art world but, at nearly 38, I had a sense that my biological clock was ticking. I knew that if I was going to get pregnant, I had to do it soon. A couple of friends told me I should wait until I was 40, but I worried that might be leaving it too late.

In the US, there's a support group for single mothers that's been going for years, called Single Mothers by Choice (SMC). I walked into their monthly meeting not knowing a soul, paid my eight dollars and was given a badge with my name on it. There were 30 or 40 women there, and we all sat down in a circle together. The meeting was led by Louise Sloan, a famous SMC who wrote a book about her experiences called *Knock Yourself Up*. Her baby boy, nine months old at the time, was there too. She gave a little introduction telling her story, and made it sound so great that I immediately thought: that's the experience I want.

Then, each woman in the circle told her story briefly; some were still thinking about becoming single mothers, some were actively trying or were pregnant and some were already parents. Most hadn't been married, but one had been married to a man who didn't want children.

I'd always wanted to have a baby, so for me, not going ahead wasn't an issue; wanting to be a mother totally overwhelmed any doubts as to whether or not I was doing the right thing. My close family were supportive. In fact, it was my mother's idea for me to go it alone, so I felt an enormous amount of encouragement before I'd even made the decision.

That said, I still had to reconcile myself to the fact that I'd be the sole parent. I thought: how am I going to explain this to my 97-year-old grandmother? For me, she was the personification of society's norms. But being in that room gave me a very positive feeling. Before, I'd thought that what I wanted to do was weird, but that first meeting opened my eyes to the fact that having a baby alone was not only a real possibility, but that it was quite normal. It gave me the strength I needed.

After the initial introductions, everyone split off into smaller groups, and I went into the 'Thinkers' group. We talked mostly about logistics: which clinics were best, the cost of transporting sperm, that kind of thing. The sperm bank with the biggest choice is in California, so a lot of people pay to have sperm shipped from there to New York. I found out that you have to decide between having an anonymous or a known identity donor too.

There were some women at the meeting who had got stuck for months at the stage of picking their donor. They wanted a nice person, but worried about how you can know that without knowing someone well. Then there were the questions of which fertility tests to have done first and who was going to pay for them. As a single woman, you go into a clinic not knowing if you have any fertility issues. And in the US, you usually have to document a year of trying before you can have tests paid for by health insurance, next to impossible if you're single.

I decided to keep things simple. So the next day, I booked an appointment at a clinic in New York that was also a sperm bank. This meant I had a much smaller selection of donors (around 40), but no transportation issues. I had to choose my donor on the clinic's website. At first, you're given brief physical descriptions of all the donors, plus information on whether they've had a documented pregnancy or not.

After that, you start paying for information. For three dollars a time, I got a longer description of the donors I might use. Then from those, I chose the three I liked best and paid 20 dollars each for a 20-page document which they filled out about themselves. These included details of facial features, hair colour, left- or right-handedness, length of fingers, educational history, illnesses, sexual partners. I was most interested in hereditary medical issues, but social ones mattered to me too; I rejected one guy because he was so into baseball and I hate it. One problem with the forms is that none of the information is checked. But I don't think there's much incentive to lie.

Some people pick characteristics of men who they'd be attracted to, but I wanted someone who looked more like me, with a fair complexion and blue eyes. My donor's hair was blond at birth, like mine. I liked the fact he was into music and played the guitar, and that he described himself as a 'logical thinker', because I am too. He said he had acne, but compared to, say, heart disease, that didn't matter to me. And I loved that he seemed very laid back; he said he was 'open to all types of foods, I like them all'. He was 21 at the time, and his SAT exam scores were on the document too. I thought they were really good – and they would have been when I took them 20 years previously. But the scoring system changed five years ago, so it turned out he wasn't quite as clever as I'd thought. I laughed when I found out.

With my donor picked, I finally started having IUI treatment. I had to travel a lot for work, which made it tricky to plan. Even the ovulation predictor tests take five minutes to tell you if you're ovulating, which is a long time to spend in the loo at work.

All my fertility test results had come back fine, so I thought I'd get pregnant on my first IUI. I didn't. My age was the only thing that was against me – the clinics prefer you to be under 35 – so I was hopeful I'd get pregnant with the second one. I'd told quite a few people I was having treatment: my mother, sister, immediate family and around 10 friends in New York. All my friends were married and none of them had had assisted pregnancies, but I still got huge amounts of support from most people, even the conservative ones.

Then came another IUI failure and another, until I'd done five in total. Until you've been there, you can't imagine what it's like. The day you find out is the day you get your period, so you're feeling pretty awful anyway. I used to allow myself one day to be angry, pissed off and upset. The whole time, there was only one day I didn't go to work, and that was because my period cramps were so bad.

I fell into a pattern. The morning after a negative test, I would tell myself: right, you've got to get up and do it again. With hindsight, I can't believe I kept going. I began to think that I'd left getting pregnant too late.

The following January, I switched to another clinic, who put me on clomiphene, an ovulation drug. I did three rounds of medicated IUI, but those didn't work either. I was lucky in one respect, that the clomiphene didn't phase me in the slightest, even though I'd read that it causes mood changes in some women. A colleague commented that I wasn't nearly as crazy as other people she'd known who were taking it. I did put on some weight, but I didn't care about that.

In April, my doctor recommended that I switch to IUI with injectable ovulation drugs – the same ones that are used in IVF. I looked at the statistics and I could see that I only had an 8 per cent chance of getting pregnant with IUI because I'd gone a year without any success. Doing the injectable drugs would take my chances back up to 18 per cent, but changing to IVF would give me a 50 per cent chance, so I decided to go straight to IVF.

I ordered the drugs, but as I was doing it through my health insurance, I had to wait a month. I was so driven that in the meantime, I did another round of IUI with clomiphene and, to do something differently, I used a new sperm donor.

It was then I decided to tell my close work colleagues that I was having treatment. I knew that IVF called for a whole different level of involvement, and I was tired of coming up with excuses for my absences. Both of them were tremendously supportive, though they were shocked to learn that I'd been trying for so long.

At first, I found the drug regime of IVF really nerve-wracking. If you're in a couple, at least there are two of you to figure out how to do the injections. That was the first time I felt angry about not having a partner. My aunt or a friend had come to a lot of my IUI appointments, so I'd never felt lost for company, but at the clinic, after the class on how to inject, I remember thinking: why can't a professional do this?

It was a steep learning curve, and I didn't always know if I was doing the injection right, especially as I had to do it at 10 p.m., when I was exhausted. Sometimes I'd be out for dinner, and have to do it in a loo. By the time I got the injection actually in my leg, I'd be so relieved.

Egg collection and embryo transfer went well: I had three embryos put back. I suspected that I might be pregnant the weekend before I had to take the pregnancy test, when I was staying with my aunt in upstate New York. I started feeling nauseous, which made me excited. Every time I went to the bathroom, I'd come back and everyone would look at me and say, 'Still got to drink orange juice?'

But the result wasn't confirmed until the following Tuesday, after a blood test first thing. That afternoon, I was in a meeting when my telephone rang. I jumped to answer it, but the clinic must have thought I was the most unexcited person in the world, as I had to keep my voice so flat in front of everyone in the office. In fact, I was ecstatic.

I told everyone who knew I was trying right away. Then, at three months, I told a lot more people, always explaining that the father was an anonymous donor. I didn't want anyone to think my pregnancy was a mistake.

At seven months, I moved to the UK to stay with Mum. I'd been given six months' maternity leave, which is very good for America, but I wasn't sure I'd be going back. And I'm very glad I moved. I'd suspected that I might need help, but I had no idea how much. Bella is now nine months old, and we're still staying with Mum for now. She has been very hands-on. We've got our own little family unit going on, and Bella gets tons of attention. Whenever my sister is here, she does bathtime, and Bella just loves my brother-in-law. She said his name before anyone else's.

I could go back to New York. But the main reason I'm staying in the UK is for Bella to have her family around her. As for my grandmother, for all my worries about telling her how I'd got pregnant, she, like everyone else, was instantly happy and surprised. Bella and I see her as much as we can; she likes to see me, but she likes to see Bella more.

As a single mum, I have to be the provider, so I'm doing some freelance work, but am also looking for a job in the UK. Eventually, I'll get my own place too.

When I look at Bella, I often wonder what about her comes from her biological father, but not in a regretful way. In fact, she looks a lot like me as a child. One day, I'll show Bella her biological father's form. The Donor Conception Network (the UK support group), says that even at her age we should be talking to her about the fact she's a donor baby. The goal is that the child should never remember when he or she was told.

All the time I was trying, I have to confess that I put all the issues about donor conception out of my mind because I couldn't even imagine being pregnant. Then, by the time I got pregnant I was so happy that I didn't give a hoot. To anyone who's using donor eggs or sperm, and saying, 'but this isn't the way we dreamed of getting pregnant', I want to say this: once you have your baby, if you had done it any other way, you wouldn't have that baby.

Q: WHAT WAS THE MOST POSITIVE THING YOU DID DURING TREATMENT?

Finding women in the same situation as me. I realised that as so many women are doing it alone, I wasn't freakish. I only went to three sessions of Single Mothers by Choice, but it was there that I met six women who I met up with for around a year. I'm still in touch with one of them. In the UK, I joined the Donor Conception Network, to meet people and so that Bella will have friends in similar situations.

Q: WHAT KIND OF SUPPORT SYSTEM DOES A SINGLE WOMAN NEED DURING TREATMENT?

I think having one or two people to come to crucial appointments – in my case an aunt and a good friend – works best. You don't want to keep introducing new people to all the various clinics and procedures. And, I suppose, one or two approximates your experience if you were going through treatment as part of a couple.

I didn't need anyone around when I got my results. I guess it depends on the type of person you are, and how you handle bad news. I like to wallow in it by myself for a day, then put on (and hopefully feel) a brave face. If you think you'd prefer to have someone there, set it up in advance – it could be even more disappointing if you are stood up. You might want to get some professional support too – for example, from a counsellor or complementary therapist. Although I had acupuncture primarily for its physical effects, I found it had a very calming effect.

Q: HOW WILL YOU TELL BELLA ABOUT BEING A DONOR CHILD?

There are generic story books that you can buy, but I'm thinking of doing a personalised photo book. You're supposed to explain it something like this: 'Mummy was very happy, but she didn't have a partner. She really wanted to be a mummy and a man did a kind thing to help her.'

You have to convey your child's conception to him or her as a positive thing. As a kid, no one wants to be different. And for a single or lesbian mother, it's more obvious when you've taken the donor route.

When a child is really young, they may not need to know everything. For example, if they ask, 'Do I have a daddy?' you can say, 'No you don't have a daddy who lives with us, but you do have a grandmother'. Then later, as they get more sophisticated, you can say, 'Yes, you do have a biological father, it's just that we don't know him'. I want Bella to know, and I don't want to lie, but I don't want her to have too much information too young. And nobody wants their three-year-old shouting out in the supermarket about semen, so you have to pick your words, like 'egg' and 'seed'.

It's hard to know how real a person to make Bella's biological dad – whether or not to say, for example, that he loves rock climbing or playing the guitar. The trouble is, if you make him into a real person, then he's a person who's not there instead of being an abstract idea.

I do have this fear that when Bella is older, a teenager, say, she's going to use this against me in some way – maybe get angry with me because I chose an anonymous donor, not one with an open identity (although she will still be able to trace her half brothers and sisters, through the sibling donor registry).

Q: WHAT'S YOUR ADVICE FOR STAYING CALM DURING TREATMENT?

In the middle of the whole experience, there were many times when I thought it wasn't going to happen. But rather than looking at the whole picture, my philosophy was to take it one step at a time. There is a lot to worry about and you'll get overwhelmed if you think about everything.

It was also important for me to have a plan, so, in this case, to know the number of cycles I was doing a certain way. That way, I wasn't going to have to wonder what to do after a failed cycle, when I was emotional or disappointed. That said, I didn't plan as much as I should have done in the beginning. I probably shouldn't have done eight IUIs, but I was afraid of having IVF, which seemed like a huge hassle and expense. Then, after eight IUIs, I thought: bring it on!

I half accepted the fact that I might not get pregnant, but my goal was to do everything I could to make it work. I didn't want to be thinking later on about what I should or could have done.

I also accepted that I was going to be stressed, then tried to minimise it. The night I was supposed to start injecting the IVF drugs, they weren't delivered on time. I could've made a stressful journey to Brooklyn to get the drugs but, after reading tons about fertility, I knew stress wasn't a good thing. So I took that month off and started again the next one. And I knew I had to look after myself; on the day I found out a treatment hadn't worked, I'd let myself be really unhappy, cry a little bit, spoil myself. I'd have the chocolate chip cookie I wanted, order in my favourite meal for dinner. But I only did that for one day. I knew I had to experience those feelings or I would have exploded later on. I allowed myself to grieve, then moved on.

• • • • • • • • •

The 2010 *Red* Annual National Fertility Report showed that more than one in four women has thought about solo parenting, and one in 20 has actually tried to get pregnant. The report also showed that the most common route to becoming a parent was to use a sperm donor, whether via a clinic or with a friend, although some women chose adoption too, either in the UK or overseas.

Amy went to meetings of Single Mothers by Choice in the US (www.singlemothersbychoice.org), but the closest equivalent in the UK is probably the Donor Conception Network (DCN.org), who run classes on becoming a parent of a donor-conceived child for both single mothers and same-sex couples. Louise Sloan's book, *Knock Yourself Up* (Avery

Trade), is a very readable account of becoming a single mother in the US. On actually being a single mother (by choice or chance) there's *The Complete Single Mother* (Adams Media Corp; see singlemother.org) by Andrea Engber and Leah Klungness.

Fertility legal specialist Natalie Gamble says it's important to be clear about your legal and financial position before you get pregnant. While sperm donation at a clinic will make you the solo parent by law, known donation or co-parenting could mean the biological father is also the legal father, even if you use a clinic. 'In many cases, it is appropriate to put in place a donor or co-parenting agreement,' she says (see www.nataliegambleassociates.com).

I'm in a
same-sex couple

· · · · · · · · · · · · ·

W
hereas families headed by a straight couple or a
single mother don't have to be public about donor
conception, a same-sex couple doesn't have that
choice. 'It's more likely that other people will know or
assume that these children are donor-conceived,' says
Marilyn Crawshaw, who leads parenting workshops for the
Donor Conception Network. 'In workshops, my experience
is that lesbian couples are much more likely to be open about
the source of how they got pregnant and committed to being
open with their children. Anything else just isn't viable,
otherwise they'd be denying their relationship.'

Some decisions are common to single women, lesbian
couples and straight couples using donor sperm, such as
whether to use a known or an anonymous donor. Going
abroad for donation can mean the child may not ever be able
to have any details of his or her father, while children in the
UK who are conceived after 2005 using donor sperm will be
able to contact their father once they reach the age of 18. But

this doesn't guarantee a positive experience, points out Erika Tranfield, co-founder of the parenting connection website Pride Angel (prideangel.com). 'And we won't actually find out the effects of this law until 2023,' she says.

Which is one of the reasons, she says, why there's been a socio-cultural shift towards lesbian couples conceiving a child with a known donor. 'These mothers want to give their child the option of meeting his or her biological father before the age of 18, so the child doesn't grow up with his or her father as an unknown in their life.' And those fathers are, often, gay men. 'Before, gay men had very few options available for them to have children. We're getting a large number of gay sperm donors coming forward, who want to play a part in a child's life.'

Erika's own family was created on this model. 'Our daughter knows her father, and sees him, but he's not considered a main parent, he's just known as Dad. She can talk about her dad at school, and that makes her no different to every other child there,' she says.

Because the law hasn't caught up with how people are now becoming parents, it can be complicated to make sure that the 'intended' parents and not the donor(s) are the legal parents. 'The most important consideration, before you start treatment, is to be aware of the law,' says Erika. 'Our site aims to provide that information so people can make their own informed decisions. There are all kinds of different rules that apply depending on whether you're using a known or an anonymous donor, and whether you are single or in a civil partnership. There are also many important decisions to be made, such as whether the donor will have financial responsibility for the child and whether he or she will be a co-parent. Don't wait until you've started having treatment to sort out your legal position.'

● ● ● ● ● ● ● ●

Harriet, 43, an osteopath from London, thought she'd left it too late to conceive.

Walking on the white sandy beach, looking at the waves, I felt an enormous sense of peace, as well as relief and lightness. I'd just had my first IUI treatment, had finally put the wheels in motion to becoming a mother. All the anxiety that comes with making an important decision had melted away, and I felt I'd done absolutely the right thing.

The clinic where I'd been treated was on the outskirts of a town called Aarhus in Denmark. It was a bright day in early spring and I could see the industrial port across the bay. It looked magical in the sunshine. It was one of those moments when you remember the details of everything: the beautiful rocks, the clean, clear water. Even though I had never met the sperm donor, I felt I was looking at where my potential child had come from.

Because I love my parents so much, the thought of having my own biological child has always been really important to me. Just before my grandmother died, when I was 28, she said to Mum and Dad: 'You must make sure Harriet has children, they're such a comfort in old age.'

But it took me until I was 39 to start trying. When I was in my 20s, my then partner, Clare, was keen for me to have children. But I said I wanted to have a career first, so I'd have enough money to support myself if anything went wrong in our relationship. Also, I'm oddly conservative at heart. When Clare and I talked about a family, we'd agreed I'd be the one to carry the baby, and I'd even looked into sperm donors. But even though my parents are very supportive of me being gay, I still wasn't sure if it was a good idea to have a baby as a gay woman. Fifteen years ago, the idea of same-sex parents wasn't so accepted, and my image of a family, which came from my own happy upbringing, included both a mother and a father.

I was also worried that Clare's family would mind her being tied down to someone else's biological child. Society doesn't seem to mind in the case of adoption or stepfathers, but I didn't think people had the same attitude when it came to lesbians.

Clare and I split up when I was in my early 30s, partly due to her disappointment that I wouldn't start a family with her. We did talk about getting back together, but didn't. She was convinced I'd never have a baby with her, and that I'd never be happy unless I had a baby.

In my life plan, I'd always intended to get pregnant at 37; I thought that by then I'd be financially secure and, in theory, it would be before my fertility became an issue. But I missed my self-imposed deadline. When I hit 38, I was no closer than I'd ever been to having a family, and I started to feel both depressed and desperate.

Although I loved my job, I'd never wanted to be a career woman. I visualised myself at home, looking after one child, perhaps two. And I didn't want to be a struggling single mum either. Becoming a mother as a gay woman is a very conscious decision. If something had gone wrong, I didn't want to be criticised for bringing it on myself.

The answer, I thought, was a male–female relationship. I started seeing men, meeting them on internet sites and going on blind dates. My mum was pleased for me; she would have preferred for me to be within the safety of a conventional relationship. I did go out with one man I liked, for about six months, but it wasn't love. I really love my parents, and I wanted to have a family in a way that they approved of, but I soon realised I couldn't fall in love with a man. I just don't connect with men in the way that other women do. Instead, I was sizing up every date as a potential father to my children. It was awful; I didn't really have any other interest in them and would always end up missing my ex, Clare, even more.

I started looking at sperm donors in the UK, but hated the thought that my child's father would be anonymous. At the time, UK sperm donors didn't have to reveal their identity to any children conceived. 'Single lesbian mother, father unknown' seemed unfair to the child and I was worried that he or she would grow up hating me for it. And I didn't want to choose a sperm donor on the basis of just a few lines of description either. I couldn't help thinking of the false claims made by my internet dates: 'tall' and 'attractive', would usually turn out to be short and decidedly homely.

So for a while, I looked for a gay man to be my baby's father. There was one candidate – a family friend. It was like a romantic proposal: we went out for dinner, and I asked him, formally, if he'd like to have a baby. He said yes, but in the end he backed out, saying he felt it would be too much responsibility. There was another man who agreed – a friend – but it didn't feel right.

In the back of my mind, I'd always wanted to get back with Clare. And if we were to have a family together, I knew she wouldn't want a third parent, the child's biological father, involved. But I still wasn't sure that Clare and I could co-parent. So, aged 39, consumed by a need to get pregnant before the age of 40, I found myself online, Googling 'sperm donors'. That's when I came across an article about Danish clinics which said that it's more culturally acceptable to be a donor in Denmark, and that lots of students do it. And, it went on, the mother can either choose an anonymous donor or one who's 'known', where you get a lot more information about him, which I wanted.

Without properly thinking it over, I looked up some Danish clinics and called one. The nurse told me to monitor my ovulation using a home kit. As soon as I ovulated, she said, I should call the clinic and book myself a flight. Unaware of a legal loophole in Denmark, where only midwives can inseminate you if you want a known donor, I'd booked myself into a doctors-only clinic. When I arrived, they told me I could only have an anonymous donor, but assured me they'd choose a lovely one on my behalf. I was desperate and, as I was ovulating and had now made the journey, I decided to go ahead.

The clinic was decorated in typical minimalist northern European style – painted white with wooden floors – and the atmosphere was very relaxed. The actual IUI process was a surprise, though, much more medical than I'd imagined. I watched the catheter going inside me and the sperm coming out into my womb on an ultrasound screen next to the bed.

A few hours later, I was walking on the beach, with a naive, romantic image that I'd conceived my much-wanted child. Neither my mum nor my sister had had any problems getting pregnant and I'd always been healthy, so I thought I would conceive that first time too. Everything just seemed right. And, two weeks later, I was pregnant. When I did the test, I had just turned 40, and I was incredibly happy.

I was still worried about bringing up a child on my own, but, as soon as I told Clare that the treatment had worked, she told me she wanted us to be together. My pregnancy seemed to solve what had kept us apart. She felt I could be happy and I could see she was happy for me.

Then, when I was 12 weeks pregnant, I started bleeding. I went to the early pregnancy unit of my local hospital, and as I was being scanned, the doctor told us it looked as if the baby had stopped growing at seven weeks. It was shocking to find out that I hadn't been properly pregnant for the last five weeks. I cried for most of that night and the next day, and Clare did too. Then, as I calmed down, my main thought was that as it had been so simple to get pregnant, I could easily do it again. And, I thought, maybe that pregnancy just wasn't meant to be.

Because of my age, Clare said I should just have IVF straight away. But I wanted to go back to Denmark and this time, use a non-anonymous donor. I booked in with the Stork Clinic, which is staffed by midwives, and chose my donor online from a sperm bank in New York that's linked with a Danish one, called Cryos. Each donor provides a written interview, including medical information, as well as more personal stuff: his favourite animal, why he wants to be a donor, a description of his family and so on. You see a picture of him as a child and, in some cases, there's a recorded interview where he talks about what's important in his life. I was looking for a man I liked – someone I wouldn't mind spending time with. Clare wasn't interested in picking a donor; she left it up to me. To her, genetics weren't important. She'd have been just as happy to adopt.

Choosing was hard. I narrowed it down to a few, and sat up one night listening to all their interviews. I could have gone for intelligence, but I didn't want a nerd. In the end, I chose a donor with a sense of humour who said he valued honesty.

The second treatment didn't work, and I began to realise that getting pregnant wasn't going to be as easy as I'd thought. Every month, I'd monitor my ovulation and, every two to three months, fly over to Denmark for treatment. I'd fly home, wait 10 days, feel myself getting tearful and know it was PMT. Four days later my period would start. I'd cry for two days, then feel more positive and start again.

I didn't mind flying over to Denmark: at least it felt as if I was doing something. And it was still cheaper than doing it in London, even with the flights, as at the time the exchange rate was very good. But after six rounds of IUI, Clare told me she hated to see me going away to Denmark so hopeful, then being so upset afterwards. She said I should switch to IVF in London. I wasn't keen: I thought it was more likely that we'd encounter prejudice in the UK, and I'd heard that some of the London clinics treat women as if they're on a production line.

By this time, the first donor's sperm had run out, so I decided to change donors. This time, I went to the European Sperm Bank (the ESB). 'Johnny' was Danish, 28 and tall, with blue eyes and blond hair, like me. I knew he was attractive to women, as he'd already got one girl pregnant naturally when he was younger. He was likeable and funny and possibly slightly irresponsible, as he was still a student. His dad was a teacher and his mum worked with children. He said that his biggest asset was that he got on with people. It made me laugh that his hobby was 'rap', as it's not something you'd think of as Danish. But I liked the fact that he seemed carefree, and that he was honest (he admitted to having smoked dope and drinking alcohol). He also liked sport, and wasn't superbly brainy. He seemed less overtly masculine than some of the others and similar to the men I get on with.

I looked at a few different clinics in London, and decided to go with Guy's and St Thomas'. Their prices were reasonable and they had good results. I had to get special permission from the HFEA (the Human Fertilisation and Embryology Authority – the body that regulates assisted reproduction in the UK) to ship the sperm to London and pay £1000 for a 'pregnancy slot', which limits the number of pregnancies in the UK from that donor to ten.

I still wasn't keen on IVF, so decided to try IUI again. It was much nicer going to the clinic with Clare than being alone. I had assumed the doctors and nurses might be judgmental about us as a gay couple, but that wasn't the case.

I had a few reasons for avoiding IVF so long. For one thing, as an osteopath, I believe in natural medicine. Also, I have always had bad PMT with lots of pain and mood swings, and

I thought IVF might make that worse. Plus, I have a benign tumour on my pituitary gland, where a lot of key hormones are produced. When your hormones are down-regulated during IVF (this means switching off your own reproductive hormones using drugs – in effect, putting you into a chemical menopause), it's the pituitary that's shut down, and I was nervous about that. But after two failed IUIs at Guy's, it became obvious that IVF was really our only option.

We discussed treatment with the consultant, and I said I would prefer to have mild IVF, where you're not down-regulated and are given smaller doses of the stimulation drugs. We were pleased with my first cycle, particularly considering that, by this time, I was 41. I got 12 eggs, nine of them fertilised, and there were three embryos to put back on day three. But I didn't get pregnant. The consultant said it was probably simply down to my age and egg quality. She said that, at 41, finding the good eggs that I had left was a bit like playing Russian roulette.

By the third failure, and now aged 42, I was starting to panic. My response to the drugs was good for my age and the last two cycles I'd even had blastocysts to put back. I kept thinking: what if I've been stupid and left it too late? Looking at the statistics, I could see that at 43, the chances of IVF working nose-dived. I even went online and started looking at egg donation in the US. Suddenly, this began to seem like a real option, even though it could cost up to £30,000.

I then decided to try and find my own egg donor, informally. I advertised on Gumtree.com, saying 'generous expenses paid', even though I knew egg donation cannot legally be a financial transaction. The ad was only up for a day before Gumtree wrote to me, saying they'd removed it 'as it isn't a job'; but I still got 40 responses.

A lot of the women who replied were impressive, intelligent and well-meaning. The majority were students, but the one I would have chosen was 24 and had just lost her job in marketing. The idea was that we'd use a donated egg and that my brother would be the sperm donor, so the baby would still be biologically related to me. The clinic agreed to do the treatment, but everybody else I spoke to said it was weird. And although my brother agreed at first, he changed his mind after his wife said she thought it would be strange for their own children later on.

Before my fourth IVF, the consultant suggested that a hysteroscopy, where the doctor puts a camera in your womb to look for polyps or adhesions, anything that could be preventing implantation, might up my chances. She also told me to take low-dose aspirin, which can improve blood flow to the womb. Meanwhile, I started to read up on other things that might help. I asked the consultant if I could go on the lowest dose of stimulation drugs possible: I'd read that this can be better for older women, and she agreed.

Around the same time, I found a book called *Is Your Body Baby-Friendly?: Unexplained Infertility, Miscarriage and IVF Failure Explained* and stayed up all night reading it, thinking I might finally have found my answer. The author of the book, Dr Alan Beer, is the US doctor who developed reproductive immunology. His theory is that a lot of failed IVF cycles are due to the mother's immune system stopping the embryo implanting. The most basic of reproductive immunology treatments is a commonly used steroid called prednisolone. Most doctors in the UK say there isn't enough proof for Dr Beer's theories, and that included my consultant, who refused to prescribe it. I then went to a private GP, but he also refused. Desperate, I ordered some prednisolone online from China, but Clare wouldn't let me take it, quite rightly saying it could be fake.

Finally, I went to see the endocrinologist who treats me for my pituitary gland problem. I took the book with me, and explained my situation. She looked at the evidence, said that in her opinion prednisolone is a safe treatment, and agreed to prescribe it. This time, I finally got pregnant. I think the steroid did help, but I assume my IVF consultant would say it didn't.

A year on, and baby Georgia is the centre of attention in our house. Once you're holding a baby, you easily forget all the awful times you had when you didn't know if that would happen. Clare is the best partner I ever could have hoped for, and the best co-parent. We've got a cottage in a little village in the country, and everyone there is so pleased for us too. Things have changed a lot in 15 years in that respect. I'm so glad I didn't end up getting pregnant with an internet date.

Q: WHAT'S YOUR ADVICE ON CHOOSING A SPERM DONOR?

Find a bank that gives you as much information about the donor as possible. In the end, I chose the ESB because they give you a written and recorded interview with the donor, a staff impression of the donor, a childhood photo, psychometric test results and an extensive family history. Details also include the known medical records, jobs and the personalities of the donor's family.

If money is an issue, look at the prices of various sperm-bank services. Exchange rates make a difference too: the ESB has a Danish and a US website.

Also, ask for the sperm count and quality on the batch you are being sent as, in my experience, they vary a lot. I didn't find out that one batch wasn't brilliant until I had used most of it for IUI. The midwife who told me also said that sometimes a woman isn't compatible with a particular donor's sperm, so it's worth trying more than one donor.

Q: DO ANY COUNTRIES HAVE ADVANTAGES WHEN IT COMES TO DONORS?

If you want a known donor who the child can contact at the age of 18, then Denmark is smaller and more accessible than the USA. I also read that it is socially more acceptable to donate sperm in Denmark, so I thought men there might be more likely to do it for the right reasons. I also preferred Denmark to the US because it has a lower crime rate and the general political feeling is forward thinking and liberal. And when I looked through the lists of US donors there seemed to be a lot more who suffered from depression and had taken Prozac. Of course, this is all my opinion, not fact.

Q: WHAT WILL YOU TELL YOUR DAUGHTER ABOUT HER CONCEPTION?

I will always be completely honest with her. I have heard that it's not being told the truth that children find hardest to accept, and which can lead to them feeling betrayed. Same-sex couples who use donors pretty much always have to be honest, in any case, as there's no other way to explain how they had children.

I will tell her that we wanted to have her and that we needed help because you need a man to make a baby, and that a kind man in Denmark helped us, and some other families in the UK, to have children. I'm going to make sure that my child will meet other donor children, which will help her to feel that she's not unusual.

Q: DID YOU ENCOUNTER ANY PREJUDICE WHILE HAVING TREATMENT?

No, none. Though one doctor did say that not so long ago, some of the older consultant obstetricians would have choked at the thought of treating gay women for fertility. Perhaps there were some medical staff I came across who did think that what I was doing was wrong, but said nothing. But I don't care because if that's true, they did a great job of hiding it. And there were enough people who were genuinely supportive to make me feel I was doing the right thing.

· · · · · · · · ·

There's a boom in same-sex parenting, but the legal situation hasn't caught up with the reality of what people are doing. To find out more about the legal issues surrounding donor conception and same-sex couples, there's a very comprehensive guide on the website of Pride Angel (prideangel.com) compiled by leading fertility solicitors Natalie Gamble Associates (their website, also with legal information, is at www.nataliegambleassociates.com). Pride Angel's primary function is to connect would-be donors and parents.

L Group Families (Lgroupfamilies.org.uk) runs workshops and meetings for potential lesbian parents. And the Donor Conception Network is excellent for advice on the emotional and practical issues surrounding donor conception. They run regular Preparation for Donor Conception Workshops (www.donor-conception-network.org). The first fertility clinic aimed at gay people has been set up in Birmingham – The Gay Family Web Centre (gayfamilyweb.co.uk). The London Women's Clinic runs the Alternative Families Show (alternativefamiliesshow.com and londonwomensclinic.com).

Stonewall has produced a guide to becoming a father (see 'A Guide For Gay Dads' at stonewall.org.uk/gaydads) with information on legal and practical issues of adoption, surrogacy, co-parenting and surrogacy. Tony and Barrie Drew-Barlow – experienced parents via surrogacy – have set up the British Surrogacy Centre to connect UK couples with egg donors and US surrogates (britishsurrogacycentre.com).

Making the right choices

• • • • • • • • • • • • •

'In every other area of your life you plan and prepare for events, and that's really worth doing with IVF because it has such a high financial, physical and emotional cost.'

'Do literally everything by the book, so you don't have any regrets. IVF is a serious medical procedure with side effects, so you need to listen to your doctor.'

'I'm not sure I would ever have held our child if we hadn't changed clinics.'

'For the last three or four IVF attempts, I'd felt that I should stop, but I couldn't face the reality of being childless. Going overseas for egg donation began to seem like a good option, if not my only one.'

How I found
the right clinic

• • • • • • • • • • • •

I VF is special because there aren't any other areas of medicine – or life – where you pay out such a large amount of money for such a small chance of success. 'Preparation is crucial,' says fertility expert Zita West. 'In every other area of your life you plan and prepare for events, and that's really worth doing with IVF because it has such a high financial, physical and emotional cost.' And that includes picking the right clinic.

Although first-time fertility patients are more likely to use their closest clinic or the one recommended by their doctor, the more cycles you have, the more likely you are to shop around.

But how do you find out which clinic is the best for you? The HFEA is against the idea of 'league tables' of results. It says clinics can't be directly compared with each other because of the variety of reasons why their patients may have had IVF, the age of their patients and the number of cycles the clinic performs. The HFEA has tried to make the statistics more understandable by stating whether a clinic's rate is above, below or within the national average. But the clinic results section of their website still makes for complicated reading.

Most clinics do come within the national average. 'There isn't a massive amount of difference between clinics, except maybe between those at the very bottom and top,' says Clare Lewis-Jones, Chief Executive of the patient support group, Infertility Network UK. She advises: 'When you're weighing up clinics, you need to ask yourself these questions. Are you happy to travel for treatment? And, what is your cause of infertility? If the HFEA figures show a clinic is doing a high percentage of, for example, male-factor cases, is it something they specialise in? And, very importantly, what is your age? Female age is going to impact on success rates. If a clinic specialises in the older patient, their average success rate is possibly going to be lower than a clinic which may only take younger patients, but it doesn't mean they are a less successful clinic overall.'

Once you've got your choice down to two or three clinics, a visit and, if you can afford it, a consultation will be useful. 'Do you like the atmosphere? Are the clinic staff understanding? All these things are important as the wrong clinic for you can make IVF more stressful – and you don't need any added stress,' says Lewis-Jones.

● ● ● ● ● ● ● ●

Sarah, 32, a pharmacy technician dispenser from Leicestershire, had radically different experiences of IVF treatment at two clinics.

My experiences of our first and second cycles of IVF were as different as night and day. The first time, my husband Duncan and I found IVF confusing, frustrating and depressing. I know the fact that the second one worked has probably coloured our judgment somewhat, and that the first cycle is always going to be a learning curve, but whereas during the first cycle we always felt in the dark about what was going on, during the second we felt informed and looked after.

We didn't know, at first, that there was a choice of clinics. It wasn't that we weren't taking IVF seriously, we just didn't realise that each clinic is different. So we decided to go to the most convenient clinic, the one closest to where we work, reasoning that it would make all the appointments easier to juggle.

It was only when I started looking at the Fertility Friends website, and saw each clinic's results on the HFEA website, that I realised there was such a variation. But I'm not sure I would have understood all the statistics at first, in any case: those rows of figures that show all the clinics' success rates are, at best, baffling when you start treatment.

We were told that ICSI was our best option, mainly because Duncan's sperm count wasn't very high and his sperm had low motility. Blood tests showed my hormones were fine, even though my cycle ranges from 25 to 40 days. Because of that, we had to wait for the right time to start treatment. That added an extra level of stress, especially as I couldn't plan ahead to book the right time off work.

At our first clinic, which was part of an NHS hospital, they put me on what we later learned was the long protocol, where you first down-regulate into a chemical menopause, then start on the injections that stimulate your ovaries to produce eggs. I ended up down-regulating for five weeks, nearly double the time that people normally do. When I came to do my first stimulation injection, I'd read the leaflets I was given, and watched the instructions DVD. But nobody had showed me exactly where in my stomach or legs the needle should go. I felt like a complete idiot, having to ask, 'Where do I actually inject?' I work in a pharmacy, so needles and drugs aren't as scary for me as they are for some people, but I still needed guidance. Once I'd got the hang of them, the injections were easy.

Disappointingly, I grew just six follicles. We felt even worse when we had a phone call from the embryologist after egg collection to say they'd only been able to collect three eggs from them.

Even before the egg collection, I'd started to lose confidence in the clinic, feeling I wasn't being looked after. A few times, I'd turned up for appointments, only to find that they had no record of them, even though I had them written down on a piece of paper the clinic had given me. Also, before the operation, I'd had to sign a consent form; I always read the small print and saw that I should have been given a particular document to read first. When I asked for the document, the nurse marched me in to see the doctor, and said, 'She won't sign the form until she sees this.' He just told her to give me the document.

At the clinic, all the consultations were done behind curtains and, while I didn't mind other people hearing about our business, I didn't like hearing that another couple had had eight eggs collected, while we only had three. It added to my insecurity.

The day after egg collection, we found out that only one embryo had fertilised. And the day after that, we had our single, only embryo put back in. Afterwards, a nurse asked me, 'So how many did you have put back in, then?' That was upsetting too. If she'd only taken the time to look at my notes, she'd have realised that we didn't have an option.

I went straight back to work the next day. I only found out afterwards that some doctors recommend rest after transfer. Maybe sitting at home would have made the difference, maybe it wouldn't. But it would have been nice to have been told that some people think it's a good idea, so we could have made the choice.

Ten days later, I started to bleed and called the clinic. I asked, hopefully, 'Could it be implantation bleeding?' and 'Will lying at home make a difference, or am I ok going to work and sitting in a chair?' In my mind, I was trying to think of the slightest thing that might help it to work. The nurse told me it was really up to me to decide what was best. To me, her voice sounded as if she thought it was all over.

By the time I had to take the test, three days later, I was resigned to the fact that the treatment hadn't worked. I had been bleeding constantly and had seen the blood every time I went to the toilet, so the failure was real for me. But Duncan still believed it might have worked. We took a urine sample into the clinic together, to take a pregnancy test, and a nurse took it out of the room to test it. When she came back in, the result was obvious by the look on her face. She said, 'I'm really sorry, it's negative. You can sit in here as long as you need.'

I didn't feel there had been much point in us going to the clinic for the test at all. I desperately wanted to be at home. I was still using progesterone pessaries and, it sounds daft now, but I didn't know if I should stop them. I had to go and hunt for a nurse to ask what to do, which made me feel even worse.

Duncan didn't say anything at all, but he drove home like a madman. At home, he was so upset, he went and lay on our bed for the rest of the afternoon. Because we'd been doing so much; injections, blood tests, hospital appointments, he'd had a lot of hope. I discovered later that, when he'd taken in one of his samples to the clinic, he'd asked about counselling, and was told it wasn't worth doing. That made me very angry. It's a big thing for someone to ask for help, particularly a man.

That's when we started researching clinics. We decided we definitely wanted to do one more cycle because everything I read said that the first cycle is a learning curve, where the doctors find out how you react to the drugs. We felt that if we didn't do a second cycle, all that information would go to waste.

I thought I had dealt with the first treatment not working, but started to realise I hadn't. I tried sitting and thinking through what had happened, but that didn't help. So I decided to write a letter to say goodbye to what we had lost. I had read about people doing this after a miscarriage. It sounds daft, but even though the embryo didn't even make it to implantation, it could have been our baby. To us, it was real and concrete. Putting everything in writing helped me to move on. I wrote: 'I feel the need to say goodbye to my last cycle before I start the next one. We both had such hope that our little embryo was going to sit snugly and grow strong inside me for nine months. Even though I have never been pregnant, this just felt so real and possible to us both. I can still see the picture of my embryo when I close my eyes. I think what I am trying to do is let go of this image before starting again.'

Before we could start our next cycle, I had to wait for my period to arrive, yet again. The timing was crucial, as we wanted to start in January, so I didn't want my period to come before Christmas, as it would have been too difficult to have time off work. In the meantime, I had to organise lots of appointments for blood tests to check my hormones before I could start the next cycle, and there was Duncan's frozen sperm to transport from the first clinic. It was like the fortnight from hell doing all that, with Christmas hanging over my head like a huge neon sign, reading, 'Sort everything out or no January cycle'.

Our second clinic, Care in Nottingham, was very different. It was much more comfortable, with places where you could sit and be quiet on your own and proper consultation rooms with doors. The staff were helpful, and went out of their way to answer my questions. It's true that it was also less stressful because we knew what to expect, and because the cycle went more smoothly. This time, I was put on the short antagonist protocol, where you go straight into injecting stimulation drugs while doing another injection to stop you ovulating too soon. This time, I produced 12 follicles, they collected 11 eggs, and 10 of them fertilised. Because it was my second cycle, I was allowed to have two embryos put back in.

Duncan wouldn't come into the embryo transfer at the first clinic at all because medical procedures make him feel nauseous. But the second time around, the staff managed to persuade him to come into theatre to see the embryos on the screen before they were transferred, telling him he might regret it if he didn't. They were really considerate and made sure there were no surgical instruments or equipment around that could spook him. All their effort really made our experience special. Duncan took a photo of the embryos on the screen, and seeing them afterwards – even though they're just black and white blobs – helped me visualise that they could become our baby.

I was much more positive during this two-week wait because the cycle had gone better the whole way through, and my breasts were uncomfortable. But Duncan refused to believe it had worked. He told himself it had failed, to protect himself from a crash if it didn't.

This time, we were told to do a pregnancy test at home, first thing in the morning. The clinic gave me one stick test to pee on and I bought a Clearblue one too, the kind that says 'Pregnant' or 'Not pregnant'. By the time I'd done the second test, the first one already showed the result as positive.

We went back to bed and lay there for what must have been at least half an hour. I don't think we knew what to do with ourselves. We'd both taken the day off, thinking it might be a negative result like the last time. We kept thinking someone would tell us we'd got the result wrong. I even took a picture of the sticks, in case the results disappeared. I think we were in shock, because we'd waited seven years for this to happen. After all the treatment, I couldn't help but think something was going to go wrong.

In fact, it wasn't until the 20-week scan that I finally started to let myself get excited that this baby was real. That's when we found out we were having a boy too. But we didn't mind what sex the baby would be – I don't think you do, when you've been through so much to get there.

Samuel was born 12 days late, a gorgeous baby. It was the weirdest feeling, lying in bed, holding him for the first time. Even though the second clinic was double the price of the first, I'm glad we made the decision to go with them. I'm not sure I would ever have held our child if we hadn't changed clinics. And now, the money really doesn't matter.

Q: WHAT DO YOU THINK MATTERS MOST WHEN YOU'RE CHOOSING A CLINIC?

You need to visit all the clinics you're considering to get a feel for them, especially the staff. When we did our first cycle, we just went for the closest one, but when we chose the second, Care in Nottingham, we weighed up all the pros and cons. It was double the price, but after our visit, we felt we'd also get double the care.

At the first clinic, everyone started injecting on a Tuesday, had their eggs collected on a Monday and the embryos were put back in on the Wednesday. To me, that doesn't seem right. I think that the cycle should follow your body, not the clinic schedule. Once we started to learn more, it was important for us to find a clinic that tailored its treatment to suit each person.

Because Duncan is nervous of hospitals and medical procedures the first clinic, which was in a big hospital, didn't suit him at all. There was only one room for the men to do samples, and sometimes there would be people outside in the waiting area, so Duncan had to produce all his samples at home and take them to the clinic. And he had to hand them to a nurse too! It was different at the second clinic; he just had to put it through a hatch and press a bell to tell the staff it was ready.

For me, it was so important that the staff had a caring attitude, and that I had confidence in them. At the first clinic, one doctor couldn't find my right ovary during my first internal scan. The nurse had to point out where to look. Lying there, legs wide apart, I was feeling vulnerable enough without feeling the doctor was still learning. In contrast, at our first appointment at Care, the consultant was very thorough, going through all the treatment we'd had and the basics of what they'd do at the clinic: the protocol, the drugs, the risks. Before that, we never even knew there were different protocols. He also put everything he told us in writing, which was helpful so I could refer to it if I had a question.

Q: DID YOU USE THE INTERNET TO DO YOUR RESEARCH?

Yes, a lot. Sometimes it was useful, and at other times it made things more confusing. When you go to the GP to have, say, your blood pressure checked, there is a precise scale to work it out on, but IVF is not an exact science. During our first cycle, our doctor would tell us, for example, our blood results, or the size of the growing follicles, but he didn't tell us whether those numbers were good, bad or indifferent.

The real problem is that it's easy to go away and start researching on your own, and frighten yourself in so doing, particularly as you've got so many new things going through your mind. I remember reading a post from a woman who was panicking because her beta hCG levels were so different from another woman's. But they were a couple of weeks apart in their pregnancies, which explained the difference. Also, different clinics use different drugs, depending on the doctor and your specific situation, so you can't judge what you're taking by what other people who are online are taking. What you need is a contact at your clinic who is happy to answer all your questions, however big, small or silly they may seem.

Q: WHO DID YOU TELL ABOUT HAVING IVF?

The thing about telling people about infertility is that while on some days you're able to talk, on others, all you're going to do is burst into tears. We decided not to tell our families. Our child was going to be Duncan's parents' first grandchild, and I didn't want to have to console anyone else if it didn't work. I don't know if I could have coped with the worry of telling them about the first failure; it just would have added more stress on top of everything else. I did tell some friends at work, and that helped day to day.

• • • • • • • • •

Infertility Network UK produce a factsheet on choosing clinics. They do ask for you to become a member, but for a small fee membership is fantastic value; there is an advice line (0800 008 7464), they campaign for fairer access to NHS treatment, put forward the patient's view to the government and work with clinics to improve their services.

Sadly, there is very patchy access to NHS IVF in some areas of the country, and none at all in others. Where you live and whether you fit your area's criteria will make the difference as to whether you will be allowed one, two, three or no free cycles of IVF. Along with other treatments deemed to be 'non-essential', it seems to be one of the first casualties of cuts. If you have been refused funding or your local authority has withdrawn funding, you should go to the Infertility Network UK website Funding For Fertility (fundingforfertility.co.uk) to find out how to appeal (the website includes sample letters and where to send them). For an interesting take on the argument in favour of NHS IVF, read Zoe Williams' article in the *Guardian* at www.guardian.co.uk/commentisfree/2010/dec/09/infertile-undeserving-ill-ivf. 'It seems peculiarly unfair to axe temporarily one of the few treatments that has a demonstrable and well-known time limit,' she says.

It seems that the future is likely to be more about self-funding. But that might not mean fewer people have IVF. The 2009 *Red* Annual National Fertility Report revealed that 95 per cent of women would cut down on all aspects of their lives from holidays, eating out and buying clothes to pensions, savings and health insurance in order to fund fertility treatment.

Having IVF
at 40+

• • • • • • • • • • • • •

Waiting in the IVF clinic when I was having treatment, one of my ways of passing the time was to consider whether the other women there were older or younger than me. After all, every year counts when it comes to IVF. According to HFEA statistics (from 2008), at 37, your chance of taking home a baby is just under 28 per cent. By 41, the age I was for my last treatment, it's 12.5 per cent. And by 43, it's 3.4 per cent.

When you go for a consultation at a clinic for the first time, it doesn't matter that you can still fit into the size-12 jeans that you've had since your 20s or that you can run faster than you could aged 16. While you've been busy living, your ovaries have been steadily ageing.

There is a theory that as your ovarian reserve reduces, the amount of drugs used in IVF should reduce too. Dr Geeta Nargund, Medical Director of Create Health Clinics, believes that the long protocol including 'down-regulation', when you're put into a chemical menopause before your ovaries are stimulated, doesn't suit some older women. 'Older women often have compromised ovarian function and low egg reserve,' she says. 'Ovarian suppression in the long protocol doesn't make sense because older women's ovaries are already suppressed.'

Dr Nargund also thinks that older women can respond better to a lower dose of stimulation drugs – so-called mild or soft IVF. 'There is no need to give unnecessary high-dose stimulation just because a woman is older. There is scientific evidence to show that higher doses of stimulation can compromise the quality of the egg and the lining of the womb,' she says. For women who would produce three or fewer mature follicles with high-dose stimulation, her protocol is to use natural IVF – a form of IVF using practically no drugs. 'You cannot make more eggs from ovaries with no or very few follicles,' she says.

This theory isn't universally accepted, however. Prescribing the right dose for each woman is never straightforward, according to Mr Hossam Abdalla, Clinical Director of the Lister Fertility Clinic. 'Clinicians want to use the minimal effective dose, and among us, we are moving to a consensus that less is more,' he says. 'But different doctors have different views, even within my clinic,' he says. The dose is up to each clinician's judgment, and Mr Abdulla says that clinicians don't want to go too low, and run the risk of getting a lower response. 'If, for example, a woman is 39 and on her last cycle produced six or seven eggs using a certain dose, I'd be reluctant to reduce it on the next cycle, even if I believed that a lower dose would produce the same result.'

That said, both Mr Abdulla and Dr Nargund agree that if a woman isn't going to make more than one egg, a natural cycle of IVF could give as good a chance as a stimulated one.

● ● ● ● ● ● ● ● ●

Sinéad, 43, a lecturer from London, found that having lower doses of IVF drugs gave her better results.

My fertility counsellor's room was right at the top of one of those tall Harley Street buildings, decorated with Eastern art, cosy rugs, and lit by lamplight. Sitting in an armchair, I'd been talking over my grief after a miscarriage when I was six weeks pregnant from my fourth cycle of IVF, and whether it was worth doing another cycle of IVF at my age – 43.

A few weeks before, I'd gone into the IVF clinic to collect my medication to start our fifth cycle, and I'd ended up walking out, crying. I'd tried to be brave but I was too scared of the disappointment if it didn't work, and of the possibility of losing a baby again. I knew the odds were against me: at 43, the likelihood of me taking a baby home was just over 3 per cent. Slim odds, by any standards.

Walking out of the clinic, I'd thought I was going to feel relieved, but I didn't. Instead I felt bereft, and a strong instinct to keep trying for a baby kicked in. Later, I rang the clinic and said that I did want to try again, after all. But one of the clinic doctors said she wanted me to have counselling first, just to be sure.

I knew I needed to stand back and re-evaluate, to be certain I hadn't lost sight of what was important to me. So I booked in to see a counsellor, Mollie Graneek. I told her our story: that we conceived our daughter Isla on my first cycle of IVF, four years previously. I explained that I desperately wanted Isla to have a brother or sister and that my need for a second child had, over time, become stronger.

Despite having had three failed cycles since Isla, which had left me disappointed and sad, I said I still wanted to keep trying. 'You're a fighter, Sinéad,' the counsellor said. 'You fought for your first child, but you have to be prepared for the fact that this is one fight that you might not win, because you're fighting nature.'

I talked to Mollie about the fact that IVF had put a huge strain on our relationship. My husband Thomas and I were still very strong together, but it was true that our lives had been on hold for months and months while we did IVF. Was it time to stop, I wondered.

At the end of the session, just as I was standing up to leave, I asked a question that had been preying on my mind: 'Honestly, tell me, am I too old to be a mother?' Even though I don't look 43, I am, and I had begun to think, if something was wrong with the baby, would people say it was my fault? Would I be the oldest mum at the school gates? The counsellor said, 'Do *you* think you're too old?' I thought about it and replied, 'No.' And she said, 'Then, no, you're not too old, Sinéad.'

There's no doubt I would have liked to have had children earlier, but I had a career and I lived in London and, like a lot of women, I didn't meet my husband until I was 37. That might be getting on in fertility years, but it's pretty normal to have a baby in your late 30s in London. Although we didn't try to get pregnant at first, we knew we wanted children. And I knew that at my age, we couldn't wait too long. So when I was booked in for keyhole surgery to investigate my painful, heavy and irregular periods, I asked the doctors to check if everything was in working order, including my tubes.

Almost the first thing the doctor told me when I woke up from the anaesthetic was that my tubes were blocked. Thomas and I knew then that I wouldn't be able to get pregnant naturally. I went back to my GP and asked for a referral to a fertility specialist, which took three months. At the hospital, the doctor actually asked me, 'Why didn't you try sooner?' And then he told me that I'd have to wait a year just to have a scan. 'A year?' I said. 'I'll be over 40 in a year.'

My GP then referred me to another hospital, St George's, where I saw Dr Geeta Nargund, a consultant there. She was very straightforward, which I really appreciated. She confirmed that I did need IVF, but said that the waiting list on the NHS was two years. She described what happens to female fertility and egg reserves – basically they plummet after 35 – and told me that I didn't have two years to wait. I looked into a few different IVF clinics then, but liked Geeta so much that I decided to go to her private clinic, Create Health.

Geeta is a pioneer in 'soft' or 'mild' IVF, using lower doses of drugs. She explained to me that she believes it's better to use fewer drugs in IVF across the board, firstly because there's less risk of serious side effects such as ovarian hyper-stimulation, but also the usual side effects, such as head-aches, bloatedness and mood swings are less likely too. Her argument is that – especially in older women – success doesn't depend on the quantity of eggs but their quality; you can make a woman produce more eggs with more drugs, but a lot of them won't be of good quality, so won't go on to fertilise.

I used to be a nurse, and I now teach nurses clinical neuro-science, so I've got a good medical grounding. Having fewer drugs fitted in with my understanding of how the body works. It made sense to me: if you think about what happens natu-rally, every month you produce one egg, and that's all you actually need.

When Geeta explained that because I'd be having lower doses of drugs the treatment would be cheaper too, that helped me make up my mind. Money was an issue for us, as we don't have a lot of it.

The first cycle was a complete breeze; no side effects, not even tiredness. I produced eight eggs, five fertilised and Geeta transferred two embryos. And we were lucky: I got pregnant, and that was our daughter, Isla.

Because of my age, we probably should have tried for our second child earlier, but my first year of motherhood was pretty full on. It wasn't until Isla started to lose her babyness, around the age of two, that I became broody and thought: Oh my God, I've got to do this again.

I'd been pretty laid back during my first cycle, but the second time was completely different because I knew what having a baby meant. I did wonder if I was being greedy, wanting another baby. But then I thought: well, it's natural to want children. And it wasn't just for me; it was for Isla. She'd started asking for a brother or sister as soon as she could talk. She carries a doll around with her, and calls it her sister. And just the other day, she said, 'Mummy, I don't want this pretend doll sister any more. I want a real one.'

I never wanted Isla to be an only child. I am very close to my own brothers and sisters. My mum died when we were very young, and we've all supported each other through difficult times, and still do. My sisters helped me through IVF. And I wanted Isla to have that support when she's older too. Being Irish, I grew up surrounded by big families. One of my best friends was from a family of nine. But those were very different times. Now, where I live in London, everyone has two children, then they stop. I didn't see why I shouldn't have that too.

When I produced fewer eggs on my second cycle, and didn't get pregnant, Geeta thought it might be worth increasing the dose of stimulating drugs slightly on my third cycle to see how I responded. But with the higher dose, I actually got the fewest eggs that I've ever got, just two. I also felt terrible physically: I had headaches and felt exhausted. And I didn't get pregnant.

For the fourth cycle, Geeta switched me to modified natural IVF, where you have even lower doses of drugs than mild IVF, so it's cheaper too. It follows your natural cycle, with a small dose of the stimulating drugs and an injection to stop you ovulating too soon. So it's relatively cheap and, physically, very easy. I produced three eggs, and they all went on to be grade-one embryos. And I got pregnant.

Then, at six weeks, I miscarried. Afterwards, I went through a process of grieving. I kept thinking: did I do something wrong? I'd started bleeding after I'd flown home to Ireland for a visit. Did I miscarry because I flew? Or because I carried my suitcase? My rational side knew it was nothing to do with either of those things, and that women have early miscarriages every day.

It was after the miscarriage that I tried to start another treatment, discovered I couldn't go through with it and ended up seeing the counsellor, Mollie. With her help, I decided I did want to have one last try. I knew that it was a complete shot in the dark. I was a little bit older than the last time, and the statistics were a little bit more depressing.

Geeta agreed to let me have another treatment – another modified natural cycle – on the proviso that it was my final go. She told me that it was her responsibility to advise me not to continue when my chances were so low. Although I was upset knowing it would be my last chance, I appreciated her being so honest.

This time, I didn't tell even my closest friends that I was having treatment. The more treatments I had, the more I felt that people didn't understand and were thinking: what, are you doing it *again*? If it failed, I didn't want to deal with everyone else's grief and disappointment as well as my own and Thomas'. So it was easier just to do it as a family: Thomas, Isla and me; it was our journey, and I didn't have to answer to anybody else.

During treatment, I grew three eggs, but only one of them fertilised and became an embryo. I had it put back when it had just split into the two-cell stage, two days after egg collection.

It was very difficult to spend that two-week wait thinking positive thoughts. Every time I found myself being upbeat, thinking it was going to work, another part of my brain would tell me, don't be silly. I spent the whole two weeks having that debate in my head.

Even though I knew the facts and the odds, I'd still had a glimmer of hope, and felt the loss when I got a negative pregnancy test.

Afterwards, when I went to see Geeta for my follow-up consultation, we didn't even discuss trying again. Part of me wanted her to say, 'Have one more try,' but she didn't. And I wasn't going to ask; she'd been very clear before.

In some ways, it is a relief to stop. I've spent the past 18 months – and at least £10,000 – having IVF. We need to get some normality back to our lives. While we were doing IVF, I never fully relaxed. I'd think constantly about it, nagging Thomas if he had a drink and worrying if I had a glass of wine. IVF consumed me, psychologically, for the months leading up to it, the month I was doing it and the recovery period afterwards.

So I'm giving up IVF, but I'm not giving up trying to get pregnant naturally. I've never found out exactly how blocked my tubes are, and I've read about women getting pregnant with partially blocked tubes. I'm going to pretend they're fine and just keep trying. I might as well. Miracles do happen, and that hope is keeping me going for now.

But whatever happens, I'm happy. Every day, I look at Isla and how can I not be? I'm a mum, and aren't I lucky? It doesn't matter how many times over you're a mum. And I'll still be a mum when Isla is 40. For plenty of women, that might never happen. I know I could become consumed with not having a second child, but that's the wrong way to think. My mantra, which I tell myself every day is, 'Be grateful for what you have.'

Q: DID YOU FEEL MORE PRESSURE DOING IVF AFTER 40?

I didn't even think about my age until after I had Isla. It was only as each cycle failed after that, that I realised age was such a big factor. But I wouldn't discourage anyone who's over 40 from doing IVF. I kept myself going by thinking: if there is one good egg left in me, it could be a potential baby.

Q: ARE YOU HAPPY HAVING A SINGLE-CHILD FAMILY?

The counsellor gave me a book of stories about single-child families. I did find parts of it useful – particularly the fact that some people actually choose to have an only child – but it made me feel as if I had a condition. I'm starting to accept that I'll probably only ever have one child.

I think of what we sacrificed to have IVF: holidays, new clothes. We live in a flat and there were times when I thought: should we be trying to find a house with a garden for Isla? Then I'd think: I'd rather have two children than a house. It was all worth it to have the chance to try. Those things are nothing, really, compared to a child. Although now, I can concentrate on saving for a house with a garden, giving that to Isla instead of a baby.

People do jump to conclusions when you have a single child, that you're an overprotective parent and your child is spoiled. But I make sure that Isla's not spoiled. I do give her a lots of attention when I'm with her, but I think that every child deserves attention; it's the biggest gift you can give them.

If life had worked out how it is in the storybooks, I'd have loved to have had a big family. But life isn't like that for lots of people, including me.

Q: HOW DO YOU FEEL AFTER YOUR MISCARRIAGE?

It's now six months later, and I'm not over it. I find being around pregnant women hard. A good friend got pregnant when I did, and we talked about having our babies together. Now she's about to have her baby and I'm not, and I can't even see her, that's how painful it is. I feel terrible, though I know she understands how I feel. I've told her, 'It's too painful to see you, you're a living example of what I want, what I should have, and what I don't have.' When her baby is born and my due date is past, I know it will be easier.

I'm determined not to be bitter about what might have been. I don't want to give out the message to Isla that having just her isn't good enough. It is. She's a little miracle.

• • • • • • • • •

When you're over 40 and trying to conceive, fertility statistics, your risk of miscarriage and your risk of genetic abnormality all seem designed to make you give up even before you start. However, although IVF success drops drastically after 40, there is still a chance. The number of women giving birth aged 40 and over in the UK is the highest since records began, at 26,976 (2009 figures).

It's worth being proactive: every month counts. Infertility Network UK (www.infertilitynetworkuk.com) has a downloadable factsheet – 'Fertility in the Older Woman', which includes detailed recommendations for a 'rapid fertility MOT' for women aged 37 and over due to their lower chance of pregnancy. (They need, it says, 'a totally different approach and understanding than those of younger years', and 'those seeking help and their medical advisors should not be complacent about the situation'.) It's worth reading, as it's very useful to know what's best practice, and exactly what you should expect or can request from your doctor.

For a woman over 40 who ovarian reserve is low, the best chance of a successful pregnancy is using donor eggs (see pages 172–3). As there is a shortage of them in the UK, and often older couples want their family as soon as possible, there's a growing trend to go abroad – to Spain, the US, Northern Cyprus or Eastern Europe – for treatment. Be aware that in some countries, donors are still anonymous, so any resulting child won't be able to know his or her genetic heritage. In some countries, you're allowed to have three or more embryos put back, so the likelihood of twins or even triplets is high. (According to figures from the Office of National Statistics, women over 45 are more likely to give birth to multiples than any other age group – www.statistics. gov.uk/pdfdir/birth1110.pdf.) If you do go down this route, it's best to use clinics with links to UK clinics, or those that are well established with good reputations, as most countries don't regulate their fertility industry as well as the UK.

In her book on becoming a mother later in life, *Right Time Baby: The Complete Guide to Later Motherhood* (Hay House), author Claudia Spahr asks experts to advise on how to improve egg quality and natural fertility, as well as increase the chances of success at IVF as an older woman. She also considers the emotional implications of trying for a baby over 40. A great website that's full of advice is www.mothers35plus.co.uk.

Not only do older would-be mothers have a lower chance of success, a lot of them worry whether, in their 40s, they might actually be too old to become a mother. Will they be too exhausted after long nights? Will they feel different from other, younger, mothers? Will their child resent having retirement-age parents when they're in their 20s? Will people be critical of them?

Amanda, who was almost 40 when she had her daughter, says she feels older mothers are often criticised for being irresponsible or selfish. 'It makes me cross. Most of us didn't make a conscious decision to be older mothers. We are, on the whole, a community of women who are very responsible. We got educated, we worked, we paid our taxes, we ate healthily, we went to the gym, but we just didn't meet a man early enough. And the life experience and financial security we can offer children is invaluable. Someone should be sticking up for our right to have children.'

I was only allowed one embryo transferred

• • • • • • • • • • • •

I f you've been waiting to get pregnant for years, by the time you're having IVF you'll want to maximise your chances of success. To this end, twins or even triplets can seem like the best possible outcome – 'two for the price of one', people often say, or 'an instant family'.

So if your doctor tells you that you can have just one embryo transferred during IVF, you may be, understandably, angry and disappointed. Elective Single Embryo Transfer (eSET), is usually advised if you're under 37, have no previous unsuccessful cycles and if your embryos are good quality. Unlike patients, clinicians see the risks and costs of a multiple pregnancy: for the mother, it could mean a difficult pregnancy and a higher risk of miscarriage; for the babies, a higher risk of premature birth, disability or death. According to Clare Lewis-Jones, Chief Executive of Infertility Network UK, 'There are very good reasons why multiple pregnancies are not a good thing, and most are to do with the health of the child. One in every twelve twin pregnancies results in at least one baby dying or having a significant disability. I can understand that patients don't want to go through any more cycles than they have to. But what is paramount is the health of the child or children.'

Something that might make you feel better is understanding that single transfer doesn't mean a reduced chance of pregnancy. 'Putting back two embryos doesn't give you double the chance of getting pregnant than just one,' says Professor Bill Ledger, Professor of Obstetrics and Gynaecology at the University of Sheffield. 'In fact, if you have a single embryo fresh cycle, plus a frozen transfer, your chances of getting pregnant are the same as having two fresh embryos together, but without the same risks.'

However, if your IVF is NHS funded, this often doesn't cover the frozen cycle. But, according to Professor Ledger, single embryo transfer is the future. 'When freezing techniques improve, single embryo transfer will probably be recommended for almost everyone,' he says.

● ● ● ● ● ● ● ● ●

Sarah, 30, a medical sales representative from Worcestershire, was only allowed to have one embryo put back on her first round of IVF.

When I first walked into the fertility clinic waiting room, the biggest shock was that everybody looked our age. I had assumed that people who needed IVF must be career women who'd waited until their 40s to start trying for a baby. But most of the couples there looked in their early 30s.

I was 28 when a doctor first told me that I'd probably need IVF because a test showed my husband Lee's sperm count was slightly lower than average. I had been pregnant once, the year before, and had had a miscarriage at six weeks, so I thought the doctor was being far too pushy and that IVF seemed rather extreme for such a small problem. I never thought I'd actually have to have it; I honestly thought I'd get pregnant first.

At the time, three of my close friends had just got pregnant, all in the first month they tried. That year, I kept creating milestones in my mind, thinking: I'll be pregnant by my best friend's wedding, then, I'll be pregnant by Christmas, then by my birthday, then by bonfire night and so on. It was a depressing time. I was wishing my life away, month by month. It was very hard to stay upbeat, not least when I got my period. Still, every time another pregnancy was announced, Lee and I put on a brave face, laughing that we'd be next.

My doctor told me that losing weight would help improve my chances of getting pregnant – I was a size 14 at the time, and weighed 10 stone 12 pounds. Brilliant, I thought, an answer, and I got quite obsessed. I joined a slimming club and in 20 weeks lost 28 pounds. But still no pregnancy.

I really thought I was too young for IVF. And I felt a bit sorry for myself, especially as I didn't know anyone else personally who'd had a miscarriage or who'd had to have IVF. So it was very reassuring for me to to see that I wasn't the only woman under 30 in that clinic waiting room. These women are like me, I thought; they're as nervous, as scared and as uncertain as I am, and, like me, they probably don't know an awful lot about what they're signing up for.

Looking back, it's laughable how much I didn't know about IVF. My original impression of it was that I'd go to the clinic, take a drug, then they'd basically put our baby back inside me. I had no idea it would take seven weeks and involve so many opportunities for things to go wrong. So we decided to go for it without knowing how intense and gruelling it was going to be. I remember, early on, Lee was reading a leaflet, and he said to me, 'You're fine with needles, aren't you?' When I asked why, he said, 'because you'll be injecting yourself every day.'

Once we knew we were starting treatment, we did what the doctors advised, stopped drinking alcohol and ate healthily. Mum was very sweet and said she'd stop drinking too, and that we could drink lemonade together. Little things like that are really touching, aren't they? But I still felt like my life was on hold, as I was constantly refusing invitations to go out.

The first stage, down-regulation, where you're put into a chemical menopause, made me extremely emotional. I had night sweats in bed and hot flushes at unpredictable times of the day. I'd be sitting in a work sales meeting, and a hot feeling would work its way up my body until it reached my face. At our Christmas work do, I remember sitting and sweating while everybody else drank wine and had fun. Although I did tell my close friends I was having IVF, there was one baby shower that I just couldn't face as my hormones were so haywire it was very likely that I'd burst into tears.

I wanted to tell my friends and family, but the problem was that some of them didn't understand IVF. So every time I saw them, they'd ask, 'So, are you pregnant yet?' And when I told them that the success rate was around 30 per cent, they would say, 'So why are you doing it then?' And I'd have to explain that we didn't have any choice. My poor family lived through IVF with us. They knew the dates of every procedure, and all about every scan and blood test.

At first, I didn't want to tell anyone at work, but in the end, I had to, as all the scans and blood tests coincided with so many work meetings, and some of them were at short notice. Really, doing IVF is like a full-time job in itself. You feel as if you're going mad sometimes. You're exhausted, making lots of eggs when your body is only designed to make one. It doesn't seem fair: the woman goes through hell, but the man only has to masturbate into a cup. But then life isn't fair.

When I wasn't in the clinic, I was living life as if I was a pregnant woman, just without being pregnant. I couldn't drink or go out dancing or even go away for the weekend. I didn't miss the alcohol, but dreaded people's reactions to me not drinking. By the time we started IVF, we'd been married for four years. And we'd told a lot of people the first time I was pregnant. So every time I refused a drink, I felt as if people assumed I was pregnant. And that's the last thing you want when you're struggling. Something that helped both of us was using the same standard answer whenever anyone asked why we hadn't had a baby yet, or if I was pregnant. We'd say, 'Oh, it's a work in progress.'

On the first cycle, I produced 12 eggs, and we had three good embryos left on day three. Lee's sperm had improved massively, so much so that they just did IVF, where they put the sperm and eggs together rather than ICSI, where they inject the sperm into the egg. He was really pleased. I was too, although it was also confusing: if his sperm was fine, it meant we had 'unexplained infertility', rather than male-factor.

I was only allowed to have a single embryo put back. That was the clinic's policy at my age and on the first cycle. The nurse explained that there was no way around it. If we wanted to have more embryos put back, she said we'd have to go to a different clinic, though it was very likely they'd be following the exact same policy. I was disappointed, as I'd have preferred to have had two embryos put back. I knew that would give us a higher chance of success, even if only slightly. But I realised that I couldn't argue. Even though I would have been happy at the time to take the risk of of having twins, I did understand the reason behind the policy, when the nurse explained that there's a higher risk of miscarriage and early delivery with twins.

A week after transfer, I started bleeding heavily. I felt very let down and disappointed. I'd been through seven weeks of IVF, sweats, moods, injections and not going out, all for nothing. I was also feeling loads of pressure from friends and family. Everyone had been very positive, saying things like, 'I bet it'll work for you'. So many people knew, and it was extremely hard to tell them all that the treatment had failed. What was good was that I had a lot of support at the clinic. I felt as if everyone there – the embryologist, the consultants, the nurses – was on my side.

Before I started the second cycle, the doctor found a cyst on my ovary during a scan. He thought it could be due to endometriosis, which would explain why I wasn't getting pregnant. That was very worrying, as the effect of endometriosis on fertility can vary so much. I did lots of research online, and found out that you can't get a definite diagnosis without a laparoscopy, a keyhole operation to look inside your abdomen. But the clinic said our best course of action was to carry on with IVF.

I didn't think the second cycle would work at all. I was relaxed all the way through treatment, didn't think about it as much, didn't put my life on hold like before. In my mind, I was prepared to have three cycles, as we knew it was roughly a 30 per cent success rate with each one. That time, out of 12 eggs, only three fertilised. It was awful when they told me that. Because of that, I spent the next few days convinced that all the embryos were going to perish. But two did really well – a huge relief.

The time from before egg collection to transfer is like taking a huge gamble every day. What if they don't collect any eggs? What if they don't fertilise? What if the embryos don't divide? What if they stop dividing? Or slow down? I have so much respect for the embryologists; I couldn't imagine doing that job because there's so much more that can go wrong than right.

Ten days into the two-week wait, I started bleeding again. This time, it was more like spotting. Assuming it was my period, I went straight to a supermarket and bought a pregnancy test, and did it in the loo. And it came up positive, straight away. I called Lee, but he was in a meeting. He knew I was worried about the spotting, so called me from the corridor, outside the meeting. When I told him the news, he wasn't expecting it and burst into tears! A woman from accounts was walking past at the time, which he said was very embarrassing. He told me to go back into the supermarket and buy another two tests, which I did, and they were both positive too.

We told our parents straight away, and there were more tears. My parents bought us some champagne, but said maybe we shouldn't drink it until I'd had my 12-week scan. As soon as they said that, I started to worry that our celebration was premature. But it turned out not to be so. At seven weeks, Lee, Mum and I saw our baby – just a little bean – on the scan. He or she had a healthy heartbeat (cue more tears).

I had a lot of morning sickness, a bad back, tiredness and swollen ankles during pregnancy, but after two years of praying for this, I couldn't complain. We decided not to find out the baby's sex, but that didn't stop me from wondering every day. And it was the best surprise ever to have a boy. Leo is now seven weeks old – a very healthy and hungry baby, feeding every two hours. Looking after him is harder than I'd imagined, but I absolutely love it.

We would like another baby at some point, a sister or brother for Leo, but I'm hoping we won't need to have IVF again. We're going to try naturally first. It's funny, when you're in the middle of IVF, you never want to do it again. But once it's over, just like labour, you forget how bad it was.

Q: WHAT DID YOU THINK WHEN YOU WERE TOLD THE CLINIC'S POLICY TO PUT BACK ONLY ONE EMBRYO?

The clinic explained that their policy – to only put back one embryo where the woman is under 37, and it's the first cycle – is part of a nationwide drive to reduce the number of multiple pregnancies. They told us that multiple pregnancies are more risky for both the mother and the babies, and that the goal is to give you the best chance of a healthy baby.

At the time, I was annoyed. All I wanted was the best chance of getting pregnant. Twins seemed like the perfect solution – a whole family in one go. And I wouldn't have to go through IVF again, either. On our second cycle, we were allowed to have two embryos put back. But now Leo has been born I think, thank goodness one of them didn't implant.

My best friend is 30 weeks pregnant with twins, and she'll have to be induced and have the babies early because she's so big. I'm really pleased I was able to have a natural labour. If I'd had twins, I'm not sure I would have managed to breastfeed either. I really wanted to, and I'm so happy that I can. I'm already out, going to clubs and meeting other mothers, and I don't think that would have happened so early on with twins.

Even though I'm only 30, and I'm fit and healthy, I'd struggle to cope with twins. I had no idea how hard looking after one baby would be.

Q: THE RULE IN FUTURE MAY BE A SINGLE EMBRYO LIMIT ON ALL IVF. DO YOU THINK THIS IS A GOOD IDEA?

I'm not sure single embryo transfer is always fair and good for everyone – each case is individual. I know the arguments in favour – the health of the mother and baby. But the argument against it is that it's not fair to expect people to pay more for freezing spare embryos, plus more for the new cycle when the frozen embryos are put back. Always including that in an NHS cycle would help.

It's already hard to go through IVF, and having to go through it more times is even harder. Also, it would be nerve-wracking if your fresh cycle didn't work, leaving you wondering if your frozen embryo(s) would defrost properly. So before a blanket single embryo transfer policy is introduced, clinics need to be certain that the embryo they're transferring is the absolute best one. I know that growing the embryo to day 5 – blastocyst stage – helps them to tell the difference, but not everyone gets to blastocyst stage.

● ● ● ● ● ● ● ● ●

The latest target for clinics is that multiple births should be 15 per cent of births after assisted conception (the target for 2010 was 20 per cent and it was 24 per cent for 2009). And it may be that the future will be single embryo transfer for everyone, as Professor Ledger suggests.

A Canadian study published in 2011[6] looked at babies in intensive care over a two-year period, and found that 17 per cent of them were there because they were from multiple births after IVF. Six of the 75 babies died.

If you want to read the arguments explaining the reasons behind the adoption of the eSET policy, go to the website oneatatime.org.uk, where the case in favour is laid out. Also, Infertility Network UK have two factsheets you can download (infertilitynetworkuk.com). You can read the original eSET guidelines, as drawn up by the British Fertility Society (BFS, britishfertilitysociety.org.uk) and the Association of Clinical Embryologists (ACE, embryologists.org.uk) on a press release from the BFS at www.britishfertilitysociety.org.uk/news/pressrelease/08_09-SingleEmbyoGuidelines.html.

What's most convincing is that there isn't an expert body that *isn't* in favour of eSET (though individual doctors have spoken out against it – see www.ivf.net/ivf/elective-single-embryo-transfer-eset-policy-implementation-toall-uk-ivf-centres-from-2009-reality-or-myth-o3976.html).

Ovarian hyperstimulation could have killed me

● ● ● ● ● ● ● ● ● ● ●

W hat would you endure for a baby? A bloated stomach? Nausea and vomiting, stomach pains and shortness of breath? Being hospitalised, put on a drip and a pipe inserted to drain the excess fluid that's collected in your abdomen?

In ovarian hyperstimulation syndrome (OHSS), a side effect of IVF stimulation, the ovaries become very enlarged with fluid, causing abdominal pain and bloating. In mild cases, which some experts reckon at around four out of 10 IVF cycles, it can be treated by drinking more fluids and, sometimes, painkillers. In more serious cases, it disturbs the body's fluid balance and, very occasionally, it can be fatal.

It's true that the risk of severe OHSS, the kind that requires medical treatment, is very small indeed – 1–2 per cent, according to the HFEA. But a report in the *British Medical Journal* in 2011[7] produced some scary headlines, saying that OHSS caused double the deaths of abortion in a 24-year period (four deaths to two) even though there were four times as many abortions as IVF cycles.

According to Mr Tarek El-Toukhy, Consultant and Honorary Lecturer in Reproductive Medicine and Surgery at Guy's and St Thomas' Hospital NHS Foundation Trust, severe OHSS can be minimised – to under 1 per cent – by monitoring patients closely. 'It's not possible to make any medical treatment 100 per cent safe. If IVF isn't performed carefully it can cause problems, but the risks are very low.' Of course, not having treatment will prevent hyperstimulation totally, but that's never going to be popular.

Clinicians in favour of mild IVF, where fewer ovulation-stimulation drugs are used, and natural IVF, where practically no drugs are used, say this is the way forward. 'With natural IVF, there is a zero risk of OHSS. With mild IVF, the risk is significantly reduced,' says Dr Geeta Nargund, consultant gynaecologist and medical director of Create Health Clinics.

According to Mr El-Toukhy, mild IVF can be useful for patients at high risk of OHSS, but it's not suitable for everyone. 'Milder stimulation will have a lower risk of OHSS, but it will also have a lower chance of pregnancy and of freezing surplus embryos for future use. It's about getting the balance right for each patient.' His view is that identifying patients at high risk, and monitoring during IVF cycles using scans and frequent blood tests is the best approach. 'The risk factors are having polycystic ovaries, being under 38, having a low BMI, especially below 22, and producing a high number of eggs, over 20. But some women who get hyperstimulation don't have these risk factors.'

The trouble is, while early OHSS (which happens after egg collection) can be predicted by close monitoring, and prevented by adjusting drug dosages, late OHSS (which almost always happens in an IVF cycle once the woman is pregnant) can't. 'Late OHSS depends on how your body reacts to the pregnancy. This is the difficult-to-prevent type of OHSS,' says Mr El-Toukhy. This is why it's so important to listen to your clinic's OHSS warnings and be aware of the symptoms, just in case you're in that 1–2 per cent.

• • • • • • • • •

Michelle, 33, a financial advisor from Berkshire, was hospitalised with OHSS.

'You're going to be very ill,' said the nurse, as she helped me into a bed on the gynaecology ward. I asked her how long she thought I'd be in hospital, thinking she'd say a few hours. 'Seven to ten days, if you're lucky,' she said.

I didn't believe her. I felt absolutely fine, apart from a pain in my side when I lay down and some bloating. During IVF, I'd followed all the clinic's instructions on preventing OHSS to the letter. They advised me to drink two litres of water and a litre of milk a day – I did it. They told me to eat more protein, so I weighed out my food to ensure I was getting 90 grams of protein a day (a recommendation I found on the internet). So how did I end up in hospital with OHSS, on two drips and, as the nurse told me, critically ill?

I knew I was at a higher risk than most women for OHSS, as I had polycystic ovaries and produced a lot of eggs during my IVF cycle. And that was why I'd been so careful to follow the clinic's instructions.

I'd learned that I had PCOS (and, most devastating of all, that my husband Stu had poor sperm too) after our first tests at our clinic, Nuffield Health. In the consultation, the doctor explained that ICSI would be our only option. I was in floods of tears and Stu just sat, staring into space, he was so shocked. We both had to go back to work, so we had a hug and went our separate ways. A few minutes later, Stu was pulled over for speeding – even when the police officer was talking to him, he said, it wasn't registering.

For the next three days, we didn't really do anything, not even eat. We just talked and tried to come to terms with the fact that we might not be able to have children. People don't often talk about infertility because it's still taboo. We felt isolated, as if we were the only infertile couple in the world. We both wished we'd started trying earlier. I'd conceived naturally with Stuart when I was 19, but had had an early miscarriage. Then we'd wanted to build our careers, buy a house and get secure financially before we had a family.

We decided we'd start treatment straight away privately, at the same clinic where we'd had the tests. I was prescribed metformin, a drug which helps keep blood-sugar levels even in people with diabetes and PCOS, and which can restart your cycle too. The clinic had also found the bacteria E. coli in Stu's sample, which is apparently very common and can lead to zero fertilisation, so he was put on strong antibiotics in the run-up to egg and sperm collection.

Because I had PCOS, the doctors said there was a chance I'd overstimulate. While I was injecting the stimulation drugs, I was scanned every two to three days. At the first scan, I had 14 follicles. At the next scan, as the doctor counted the follicles, I started counting them on my fingers too. He said, 'You're not going to have enough fingers – or toes.' I had 31 follicles, plus a few tiny ones. But I felt fine; there was no bloating, and I was still in my size-8 jeans.

A blood test showed my oestrogen levels were high, another risk factor for overstimulation. So the doctor reduced my final dose of the stimulation injection and prescribed a drug called cabergoline. After another blood test, he said I was fine to go ahead with the final trigger injection, the one that ripens your eggs and gets them ready for collection.

The clinic warned me that the doctor wouldn't do the embryo transfer if I had any signs of OHSS. Instead, they would freeze the embryos and wait until my body had calmed down. But I was determined to have the transfer – I felt well and was sure I wasn't really at risk of OHSS. And how serious could OHSS be, in any case, I thought. I was only coping so well with the treatment because there was a chance I'd get pregnant; having to wait would have been a real blow.

After egg collection, the embryologist told us that we had 24 eggs, and, even better, that Stu's sample was bacteria-free. We were delighted and couldn't stop smiling. That weekend I still felt fine and there was more good news: 17 out of the 24 eggs had fertilised. The embryologists froze eight embryos on day one, which left us nine.

But when we came back for embryo transfer three days later, a scan showed there was a little bit of free fluid in my tummy, a warning sign of OHSS. I was still in the same jeans, so I wasn't bloated, but the doctor said he wasn't comfortable doing the transfer. He said we should wait another two days, which should give my body a chance to recover. When another scan two days later showed no sign of fluid, he decided to go ahead, transferring one embryo.

At home afterwards, I rested for a few days, watching DVDs on the sofa. I did feel bloated by then, but not uncomfortable. We decided to go to the seaside for the weekend, to Southsea in Hampshire, just over an hour's car journey away. When I got out of the car, I couldn't walk more than a few steps because my tummy suddenly felt so hard and bloated. We drove home straight away, in case I had to go to the clinic. But I felt fine for the rest of the weekend, so I put the bloating down to the progesterone pessaries I was using, and maybe doing too much too soon.

Then, on Sunday night, every time I lay down to go to sleep, I felt a shooting pain in my left shoulder, and I couldn't breathe properly. Stu said we should call the clinic straight away, but I said I was fine sitting up watching TV. I didn't want to wake up the nurse on duty until a reasonable time. At 6 a.m., I called and the nurse told me to come straight to the clinic to be scanned.

While scanning me, the first thing the nurse said was, 'I think you're pregnant,' which started both of us crying. She kept scanning, and told us I did have some free fluid in my tummy. She went into the nurses' room next door, leaving the door open, and I heard her say, 'She has got a load of fluid in there'.

The head nurse came and sat down with us. She said I had OHSS, that she was going to call the fertility unit of the local hospital, and that we should go straight to A & E. I called work to say I'd probably be in that afternoon.

In A & E, a very kind nurse came and took my details, and told me to keep drinking water. Then I had eight vials of blood taken, was put on a drip and taken up to the gynaecology ward. Settled in bed, I told Stu I felt fine, and he should head off to work. But just then, the A & E nurse came running in to tell me that one of the tests they'd done was a beta hCG test, and it was positive.

The consultant put me on a second drip, saying that the OHSS had made me very dehydrated, despite the fact that I was drinking non-stop. And the nurses started measuring the amount of fluid going in and out of me. That night, I began to swell up. When I was weighed in the morning, I'd gone from 9 stone 10 pounds to 12 stone, and the extra weight was all fluid around my middle.

I had yet another scan, and the doctor said, 'I'm really sorry, but I'm going to have to drain you.' I didn't know what he meant, so he explained they were going to insert a tube into my abdomen to get rid of the excess fluid. I was wheeled down to theatre, then given a local anaesthetic next to my hip bone. It felt like I was about to be tortured: I could see a line of sharp instruments and a tube on the table in front of me.

The nurse held my hand while they made the cut. I could feel pressure, then when the doctor pushed the tube through my stomach muscles, I heard a horrible crunching sound. He put in the tube and drained off masses of bright yellow fluid. Then he attached a bag to the tube. The bag could hold a litre, and by the time I'd been wheeled up to the ward, it was already full to bursting. The nurse emptied, then re-attached it, and it stopped filling. She said I probably didn't have any more fluid inside me, but that didn't seem right, as I was still very bloated.

In the next few hours, I blew up so big that there were tiny veins actually bursting on my tummy. Stu said it looked like someone had strapped a barrel to me. I was wearing my sister's size-22 maternity nightie and it was like a second skin.

That night, after Mum, Dad and Stu went home, was the worst of my life. My legs wouldn't work properly, and that made me scared. The skin on my stomach felt as if it was ripping. It was like I'd suddenly become nine months preg-nant overnight. I've never known pain like it; I was crying – and I'm not a crier. When a nurse came and held my hand, I remember asking her if I was going to die.

They gave me morphine, but it didn't touch the pain. Around 3 a.m., a consultant gynaecologist came up. He took off the plaster around the drain and discovered it had kinked up inside me, which is why the fluid wasn't coming out. He straightened it out, then attached a massive syringe, and started to pull the fluid out of me. He drained two litres out of me in 10 minutes.

It was an incredible relief to have some pressure released. I half passed out, half fell asleep. Between 4 and 6 a.m., I remember hearing the nurses emptying the fluid bag. When I woke up, they told me another eight litres had come out. It was the same routine for the next few days: having the bag changed, being weighed, having blood tests. The highlight of the day was when the consultant came up and told me my beta hCG result. As long as it was going up, I was still pregnant, so I knew I could get through anything.

When I had the drain taken out, 10 days later, the nurses told me they'd taken 28 litres of fluid out of me, and I'd had 37 transfusions of human albumin to correct the fluid imbalance. They showed me a consent form I'd signed when I arrived. I'd thought at the time that I was fine, but I didn't remember signing and I didn't recognise my signature, which was huge and scrawly.

Back at home, I still felt poorly, but I was happy vegging out on the sofa. A week later, at my six-week scan, it was hugely emotional when the doctor pointed out a tiny flicker, the heartbeat that told us our baby was still alive. We were overjoyed, especially considering all the drugs I'd had. Another scan at eight weeks showed everything was going well and, finally, I started to feel more confident.

Then, a week later, I was in the supermarket, and started to have the most bizarre period-like pains going down my leg, back and tummy. They lasted around an hour, although there was no bleeding.

I had booked a private scan as a birthday present to myself the next day. As soon as the doctor put the probe on my tummy, I could see there wasn't a heartbeat. I said, 'Look the heart's not flashing.' And the doctor said, 'No. I'm sorry, it's not.' Stu looked as if he was going to pass out. That night, neither of us slept much. We just sat up, waiting until morning when we could go to see my GP.

I refused to open any presents on my birthday. There was nothing to celebrate. I wanted it all to be over; I couldn't bear the thought of having a dead baby inside me.

I had the operation a couple of days later. We were both so down; it was the worst time. Later on, the consultant told me the miscarriage had had nothing to do with the OHSS or treatment, but I'm still not sure. I think I'd have been able to forget about being in hospital if the baby had been fine. But with the miscarriage, it all seemed unbearable.

We hadn't told most of our friends and family that we'd been having treatment, which made it easier, as no one asked any questions. But Stu and I were also conscious that we needed to explain why we'd been such bad friends, missing so many parties and celebrations that year. We were too upset to do it in person, so we sent an email to everyone, describing everything that had happened.

We went on holiday to Turkey, just to get away. Even though it was December, it was warm and we sat by the pool and drank cocktails. And we talked and decided to have some of our frozen embryos put back in the New Year.

The clinic thawed four of the eight. We were very nervous as to whether they'd survive, but on day three, there were still three embryos, two looking quite good. I had those put back in and off we went for another two-week wait, relieved to know there was no risk of OHSS after a frozen transfer.

I woke up at about 6 a.m. on testing day, and went to the bathroom to do the test. We were convinced it would be negative because there's less chance with a frozen transfer, and my body had been through so much. I thought I saw a pink line, which would mean it was positive, so I passed it to Stuart, and we kept passing it back and forth, feeling increasingly happy as the line got darker.

That night, we went out for pizza to celebrate; I had a bit of tummy ache, but thought nothing of it. When we got home, I went for a wee and found I was bleeding. I was absolutely petrified and called Stu in to see the blood spots in my knickers. I phoned the clinic and they told me to go straight to bed.

I carried on bleeding all day, every day for 10 days, heavily enough to soak through a pad. I made Stu come to the toilet with me to hold my hand, as I was so scared of what I'd find. At five and a half weeks pregnant, I was sure I was miscarrying, so I begged the clinic for a blood test, which they don't usually do. When the nurse called with the results, she said, 'A beta hCG level of more than 10 is pregnant. None of us can believe it – your level is 14,633!'

The following week, I went in for my six-week scan as planned, still bleeding, completely terrified. We did see a baby, and a heartbeat, but there was blood everywhere. Just two days later, I had cramping and went back in for another scan, but the baby was still hanging on in there. The doctor thought the bleeding was probably coming from the second embryo, the one that hadn't survived.

The bleeding got even worse and, when I was seven weeks pregnant, I started passing big clots. I called the hospital and was told to bring them in. The doctor thought it did look like foetal tissue. That night, I was admitted to the same ward as before, put on nil by mouth and on a drip, and told I'd have a scan in the morning. Stu and I both knew what all that meant: an operation. It was horrific.

I'd grown close to some of the nurses on the ward, and they came to see me; it was bittersweet, as they hadn't known the previous pregnancy had ended and I had to tell them this was a new pregnancy I was losing.

In the scanning room the next morning, at first the doctor turned the screen away, so I couldn't see it. And then she gasped and turned the screen back. 'There's your baby,' she said. Stu and I were overjoyed.

The bleeding lasted another two days, then I started passing white lumps. So I went back in for another scan – and the baby was still fine. The doctor said the white stuff was probably membranes from the other foetus.

I carried on having private scans every week until 14 weeks because I was so scared of having a miscarriage. It cost a fortune – £105 each time – but it was well worth it for peace of mind. I also bought a Doppler machine to listen to the baby's heartbeat when I was feeling nervous too. It wasn't until I got my maternity pay form from my midwife at 25 weeks that I relaxed.

Owen was born the day after my birthday, a year after I miscarried. And it was the doctor who'd unkinked my drain when I had OHSS who delivered him. He's only 12 weeks old, but it seems as if he's been with us for ever and I feel so lucky. What a difference a year makes.

Q: WHAT DID YOU THINK ABOUT THE RISK OF OHSS?

I was told I had a higher risk of OHSS because I had polycystic ovaries. And I was warned again at the first scan after I started the stimulation drugs because I was growing so many follicles, another risk factor. In our first consultation, the nurse had stressed that OHSS could be really serious but I think that when you're doing IVF, you are blinkered about any risks. You just assume that OHSS won't happen to you. All I wanted was to get on with having treatment and to get pregnant; I think that's the same for the other women I've spoken to who've had IVF. Unless someone told me, 'You're going to die', I would run the risk of OHSS again for the chance of having a baby.

Q: **WHAT ADVICE WOULD YOU GIVE TO ANYONE DOING IVF?**

Do literally everything by the book, so you don't have any regrets. IVF is a serious medical procedure with side effects, so you need to listen to your doctor. Both Stu and I said that if IVF didn't work, we didn't want to look back and wish we'd tried a little bit harder. So pretty much from our first clinic appointment, we cut back on processed foods and cooked everything from scratch. We both took supplements; the clinic recommended Stuart take selenium and I looked for advice online, and started taking co-enzyme Q10, royal jelly, a pregnancy multivitamin, omega 3, selenium and zinc. We stopped drinking caffeine and alcohol, and I started drinking two litres of water and a litre of milk daily straight away. I've never drunk milk, can't stand the stuff, but I drank it because it was what the clinic recommended.

Because I had polycystic ovaries, the clinic told me that the protein content of my food should be higher than the carb. I was so careful that I cut down my carb intake to tiny amounts. The clinic didn't tell me exactly how much protein to eat, but I worked around a figure I found online of 90 grams a day. Two packs of cooked chicken pieces was 60 grams, then I'd add in the milk, other meat and some cheese. I remember one day craving a cheese sandwich like nothing on earth, and I weighed it out to make sure there was more cheese than bread.

I knew that following the fluid and protein guidelines was especially important as I had PCOS. You should ask your doctor about your risk. And don't ignore symptoms like I did. Some people feel really ill with OHSS, but others, like me, don't. If you do need treatment, the sooner you get it the better.

OHSS isn't something to worry about (you've got enough to occupy your mind during IVF), but it is something to be aware of. Your clinic should be very clear about which symptoms you shouldn't ignore, and when to contact them. That said, mild hyperstimulation is extremely common. It's uncomfortable, but I found the worst thing about it was how bloated it makes your stomach, which can be embarrassing when you don't want people to assume you're pregnant.

If you have had OHSS before, you will be monitored more closely on any subsequent cycles, and may be given lower doses of stimulation drugs as well as medication to prevent it.

The NHS guide to OHSS can be found at www.nhs.uk/Conditions/Infertility/Pages/Complications.aspx. As they point out, you should seek medical attention if you have any of the symptoms, as OHSS needs clinical assessment.

I had reproductive immunology

• • • • • • • • • • •

I f there's one issue that's guaranteed to raise the hackles of fertility experts, it's reproductive immunology (RI). There's a huge divide between doctors who believe that a malfunctioning immune system is the key to many recurrent miscarriages and IVF failures and those who say the evidence isn't there.

It couldn't be more confusing for the patient. On the one hand, you hear stories of women who've had five, seven or even eleven rounds of IVF before conceiving after RI. And clinics that specialise in immunological testing and treatments, such as the Assisted Reproduction and Gynaecology Centre (ARGC) in London and Care Fertility in Nottingham, have above-average success rates.

On the other hand, prominent NHS specialists have spoken out against it. The miscarriage expert Mr Raj Rai, who wrote the opinion paper on it for the Royal College of Gynaecologists and Obstetricians (RCOG) says in the paper, 'To date, there is no convincing evidence that reproductive failure occurs as a result of immune rejection.'

Most of the original methods of diagnosis and treatment were developed in the US by a doctor called Dr Alan Beer. Dr George Ndukwe of the Zita West Assisted Fertility Clinic in London, who was mentored by Beer, was one of the first clinicians to adopt Beer's tests and treatments in the UK. He says, 'For a successful pregnancy, the woman's immune system must allow it. The only time anything foreign comes into the human body and is not rejected is pregnancy. Anything that goes wrong with this system can affect implantation.' Dr Ndukwe believes that, of IVF cycles where the embryo fails to implant, around 20 per cent – that's one in five – are down to immune issues. Of the rest, he says, 75 per cent can be blamed on the embryo being chromosomally abnormal and 5 per cent are due to uterine factors, such as endometriosis, fibroids or polyps.

The main argument against reproductive immunology is that there just aren't enough large-scale good-quality studies to prove that it works. But the studies to provide this proof would simply cost too much, according to Ndukwe, who estimates the bill would reach as much as £3 million.

The most contested aspect of this controversial topic is natural killer (NK) cells. Too many of the wrong kind, say some doctors, and the embryo can't implant or stay implanted. The establishment disagrees. 'It is not clear whether the NK cells normally found in the blood ever do attack the foetus. Or whether measuring then suppressing the level of NK cells in the blood has any effect on the chances of a successful pregnancy,' says the HFEA.

Clinics test for other possible immune problems too. There's 'allo immunity', the theory being that if a woman's biologically similar to her partner, she may not produce the correct antibodies to block the embryo from being attacked by her own immune system. Or IVF failure may be due to a high level of TNF-alpha (tumour-necrosis factor alpha), which causes the inflammatory response – and some of the nasty symptoms – in autoimmune conditions such as psoriasis, rheumatoid arthritis and inflammatory bowel disease.

At most clinics, reproductive immunology treatment will depend on your diagnosis after a blood test which is sent to the US. Treatment could be baby aspirin, a steroid called prednisolone and/or the blood-thinning drug, clexane. Or it could be much more expensive: a TNF-alpha inhibitor called HUMIRA (adalimumab), intravenous immunoglobulin (IVIg), a blood plasma product usually given to those with autoimmune conditions. A newer and cheaper replacement for IVIg, Intralipid, is an intravenous fat emulsion made from soya beans and eggs.

Mr Ndukwe says that more doctors are starting to believe that RI is valid. But, he cautions, it's important to have the tests to determine whether you need treatment, which treatment you need, and to measure whether the treatment is working.

All of this can add thousands of pounds to the cost of a cycle of IVF. There are plenty of stories – both online and in the press – of women who got pregnant afterwards (like Alice, below). The stories can seem like compelling evidence to anyone who's desperate to get pregnant – but some people simply can't afford the tests and treatment.

Mr Hossam Abdalla, Clinical Director of the Lister Fertility Clinic, which does offer reproductive immunology, thinks that immunological issues could be indicated in some cases – but perhaps not in as many as some doctors believe. 'If the patient has had three or more cycles with good embryos, and her uterus looks healthy, I would offer the test, while informing her that the science behind it isn't very clear and the treatments can be costly. That patient could be one of the few who might benefit. Although we are knowledgeable, we don't have all the knowledge. There are many other factors that cause IVF to fail that we don't yet know about. The most important thing with IVF is that, if people carry on trying, they increase their chances.'

• • • • • • • • •

Alice, 38, and her husband Alex are GPs from London. After four failed attempts at ICSI, they decided to try reproductive immunology.

Still in my pyjamas and slippers, I opened the door. I couldn't believe what I saw. It was three of my closest friends – a hospital consultant, a GP and a nurse – all togged up in full clown gear, pancake make-up, bright wigs and crazy, shiny clothes. They'd come to cheer me up during my two-week wait after embryo transfer and before my pregnancy test. I realised why one of them had sounded so odd when I'd called to ask her if she'd pick up the takeaway on the way over.

My friends got the idea to dress up as clowns from some research that had just come out, a study done in Israel. It showed an increased IVF success rate for women who had been cheered up by a clown. All night, even when we were talking about serious subjects, I kept laughing because they looked so stupid. They are adamant, to this day, that it was them who got me pregnant!

Joking aside, this was Alex's and my fifth and final cycle of IVF, so we were desperate for it to work. We'd known from early on that we'd need to have treatment, as Alex had a low sperm count of 2 million per ml (over 15 million per ml is normal). In four failed cycles, we'd only had one positive pregnancy test, a biochemical pregnancy, where the embryo started to implant but lasted a few days. So for that one cycle, we'd decided to throw everything we possibly could at it.

I spent a lot of time on the Fertility Friends website – especially on the 'poor responders' thread – asking lots of questions and reading up as much as I could. We decided to have four different treatments, addressing any factor that might possibly make a difference and help me get pregnant. It was going to bring the price of that single cycle up to around £20,000. But if we didn't go for it this last time, we thought we'd always regret not trying. I felt the most positive I'd felt so far, because I knew we were doing everything we could. At the same time, I felt relief because I knew I'd never have to go through IVF again.

I had always had very painful periods, one of the signs of endometriosis, and I suspected that might be what was stopping me from getting pregnant. My GP didn't think I had it, but he agreed to refer me privately to a consultant, who didn't think I had it either. With endometriosis, cells similar to those of the uterine lining grow outside it in your abdominal cavity. As they grow, then bleed, every month, it can cause adhesions and stop your reproductive organs from working properly.

At the moment, it's impossible to tell definitively if you have endometriosis until you're opened up. So the month before treatment, I booked in for a laparoscopy, an operation where a camera is put through an incision next to my tummy button to look for signs of endometriosis. It turned out I did have it, so during the operation the surgeon lasered away the adhesions in my abdomen that it had caused.

While I was under anaesthetic, I had a hysteroscopy too, where the surgeon put a camera inside me to check my uterine lining and cervix, and measure my uterine cavity. At my fertility clinic, the ARGC, the doctors are very much in favour of doing this, as they believe it helps to improve implantation rates.

We decided to have two controversial reproductive immunology treatments too. Some doctors worldwide believe that IVF implantation failure and multiple miscarriage can be caused by specific elements of your immune system being overactive. However, most fertility doctors in the UK don't believe there's enough proof that these treatments work – various studies have been inconclusive.

The first treatment we had, lymphocyte immununisation therapy (LIT) was at the Portland Hospital, in London. (It's based on the theory that in a normal pregnancy, your body recognises the embryo as foreign, and produces antibodies to protect it from your immune system. If your partner is biologically similar to you, the embryos aren't foreign enough, so this process doesn't happen and your body rejects the embryo.) The treatment involved me being injected with white blood cells that were taken from Alex's blood.

The other reproductive immunology treatment we had, this one during IVF, was IVIg (intravenous immunoglobulin), an intravenous treatment derived from blood plasma. The theory is that this combats high levels of natural killer (NK) immune cells, which can stop implantation and pregnancy.

We had to weigh up carefully whether to do these unproven treatments or not, but after examining all the evidence, and taking into consideration that we didn't have any other options, we were both happy to go ahead. I suppose we were lucky that, as doctors, we could understand the medical arguments more easily than most – and that we had saved enough money.

My parents, who have a scientific background, didn't want me to do IVIg because it's derived from donated blood, which means it carries a very small risk of contamination and infection. And reproductive immunology treatments don't come cheap; we spent over £5000 on those two treatments alone. But my thinking was, this is my last go; I've just to got to give myself over to the doctors and trust them.

I have no idea which of the treatments worked, but that was the cycle in which I did get pregnant. Getting the result we'd wanted for so long left me with a strange mixture of emotions: disbelief that it had finally happened, and total elation.

I didn't have the easiest pregnancy, although I loved being pregnant, and felt so lucky every day. I started bleeding early on, then, at the six-week scan, there was no heartbeat. At the same scan, they found a big blood clot next to the foetus. But a week later, there was a heartbeat.

Then, after the 20-week scan, the consultant told us the baby had a slight defect in her heart, called an echogenic focus, and two big cysts on her brain, both possible signs of genetic conditions, such as Down's syndrome or another syndrome called Edwards. I was petrified for a few days after the scan. But when looking into the results further, I discovered that very often, normal babies have these signs at 20 weeks. I found stories of people who'd had the same results, and the babies had been fine. By the scan at week 28, the worrying signs had disappeared, thank goodness.

But at 32 weeks, the baby's growth started to slow down. At 34 weeks, my urine tested positive for protein, a sign of pre-eclampsia, so I had to be admitted to hospital. With pre-eclampsia, your body begins to reject the placenta, and it's dangerous to both mother and baby. A week later, in the middle of the night, my blood pressure shot up, and I got severe pains in my liver, both signs of HELLP syndrome, which is similar to pre-eclampsia and, I knew, potentially life-threatening – for both of us. Sometimes, as a doctor, too much knowledge can be scary, and this was one of those times.

The doctor who was on call decided to induce me immediately, but then the baby got distressed and I had to be rushed into theatre for an emergency Caesarean. The delivery room was packed with people. The operation was so rushed that they couldn't get the epidural to work. I could feel them opening me up, which was incredibly painful, so they gave me a load of morphine. When Maia came out, I was so out of it that I can hardly remember it; it was more like a dream. She was small, at 4lb 9oz, but luckily, she screamed straight away and fed really well too, so she didn't have to go into the special-care baby unit. She was a gorgeous baby. I had to be monitored every 20 minutes for the next 24 hours, but we were home three days later.

We had tried for so many years to get pregnant naturally and by having IVF, so when the health visitor asked about contraception, I found it funny. Alex and I knew we wanted another child. We thought it might take years, so when Maia was six months, we went back to the clinic to book in for our next cycle of IVF. The doctor there sensibly told us to go away and enjoy Maia some more before jumping into the whole thing again.

But, the next month, I found out I'd got pregnant naturally. I hadn't even got my periods back. Alex and I were blown away with happiness. This time, it was a really easy pregnancy; I didn't even have morning sickness.

Now, three years later, we're happy with our two gorgeous girls, and feel so lucky that they are both healthy. We're out of the baby stage, I've had a coil fitted and we certainly wouldn't try for another baby. But there's one thing that preys on my mind. We have one embryo frozen at the clinic, and I can't bear the thought of letting it go. We have talked about donating it to another couple, but we were told you have to have more to do that, as there's such a high chance that a single one won't survive the thaw.

I go through phases where I'm certain I'm going to have it put back, then I think: what if there is a problem? What if the child isn't healthy? I am absolutely torn. If we hadn't been successful on that last cycle, that frozen embryo would have been my last and only hope for a baby, the most precious thing in the world to me, as we weren't going to have any more fresh cycles. Whatever I decide, Alex has said he'll support me.

We've only got a few months now before the embryo has to be destroyed. I see that embryo not as a ball of cells, but as a possible person, as Maia's twin, in fact. She's such a precious little girl and to know there's a possibility of another one like her is very tempting.

Q: WOULD YOU RECOMMEND REPRODUCTIVE IMMUNOLOGY?

It's really up to you to think about what's right for you. If you're lucky enough to be able to afford to have these extra treatments, and you've had failed cycles, and your doctor says you're a good candidate, I think they're worth considering. It's true that reproductive immunology is controversial, and that the proof isn't there. But it's also true that I don't think Maia would be here if we hadn't gone ahead, even though I can't be sure what worked as we did so many new treatments at once. But as IVF is such a big investment – in time, energy, emotions – we didn't have the luxury of doing them one by one. I decided to trust my doctors, and I knew they believed in what they were doing. Equally, if you feel uncomfortable about reproductive immunology, it may not be for you.

Q: AS A GP, A LOT OF YOUR WORK INVOLVES PREGNANCY AND BABIES. WAS THAT HARD FOR YOU?

Treating babies was absolutely fine but, at certain times, seeing a pregnant woman, a belly with a lovely baby in it, would leave me in tears. I found it easier to counsel people with fertility problems because I was in the thick of it myself, but it became much harder to sign off women for terminations. I had to ask my colleagues to take on that responsibility.

Q: DID YOU DISCUSS YOUR NEXT STEP IF ICSI DIDN'T WORK?

After three cycles, a really lovely friend, Kate, offered to be our surrogate. I was so grateful, I felt overwhelmed. It did feel a bit weird to think I might not carry my own baby. But, if it had come to it, Kate would have given us the best present anyone could ever give. She was such a great friend, she was prepared to put her life on the line for us; women can die during childbirth.

Surrogacy was our logical next step, as I always made enough eggs of good quality and we usually had enough sperm for ICSI. Kate had really enjoyed being pregnant with her own children. She thought hard about how she'd feel, carrying our baby, and decided that as it would be genetically 100 per cent ours, she felt she wouldn't have any problems handing over the baby after the birth.

The discussions got quite serious: Alex and I went out for dinner with Kate and her husband and talked about the legal and practical implications. They're a very family-oriented couple and they knew how desperate and sad we were, and could see we'd make good parents. But there was one major issue: they hadn't yet finished their own family. They had two children and wanted a third in around a year, so we would have had to wait for quite a long time. And it turned out that Kate had lots of health problems in her third pregnancy, so it's lucky we didn't need her in the end.

By the time we got to our fifth cycle, Adam was very happy to stop treatment and to adopt, but I really wanted to give it one more go. I craved a biological attachment to a baby, and to be pregnant and to give birth. I was prepared to adopt, but I honestly think I would have always wished that I'd been able to carry our baby.

Q: AS A MEDICAL PROFESSIONAL, DID YOU SEE A LOT OF MISTAKES AND MISCONCEPTIONS ON THE ONLINE FERTILITY FORUMS?

The trouble is, there's no regulation, and a lot of the information is hearsay. There is some misinformation, but I didn't see anything actually harmful. If someone posted information that was badly wrong, especially when it came to medication, I always posted to correct it.

For me, the forums were most useful to find out more about the alternative side of fertility, that's not based in research but more on anecdotal evidence. I'm not saying that complementary therapies definitely make a difference, but at least you feel like you're doing something and, I think, psychologically that's really important.

Q: HOW SHOULD PEOPLE JUDGE WHICH COMPLEMENTARY THERAPIES ARE RIGHT FOR THEM?

You've got to be comfortable with any therapy, to feel positive about it and believe it will change things. Reputable therapies, like acupuncture, will usually have a central organisation that can provide you with some kind of evidence or explanation of how it works. Look into the evidence, talk to friends and go on forums to see what other people are doing. The problem is that there isn't enough research so, like I did, sometimes you have to trust your instinct.

I liked acupuncture, and found it calming. My husband went to see a Chinese medical herbalist too; we made sure it was a clinic with a good reputation, as there have been problems with some Chinese medicines being contaminated.

I also had a fertility hypnotherapy CD, which I listened to when I needed to relax. But when I went for an appointment with a hypnotherapist, I hated it. At first, I lay down, and it was nice and warm, and I felt very sleepy. But when the therapist started the hypnosis part of the treatment, she just sounded really bored, as if it was the hundredth time she'd done it that day. It cost over £100, so I didn't go back.

Q: WHO HELPED THE MOST WHILE YOU WERE TRYING TO GET PREGNANT?

The women I met online, through Fertility Friends. Friends with kids had all got pregnant relatively easily and they were all very supportive and lovely, but it was hard as they didn't totally understand. People try to help, but they just have no idea. They'd say things like, 'Don't worry, it'll happen', when you really don't know if it will or, 'Adoption isn't that bad'. And someone once said, 'I know how you feel, it took me four weeks to get pregnant,' which was pretty unhelpful.

In the forums, people understood because they'd had the disappointment of a negative pregnancy test themselves and knew how it leaves you feeling so hollow and horrible. I'd go on the site every day, and sometimes groups of online friends would meet up too. Once, when Maia was eight months old, 20 of us met at a pizza restaurant in London. It was like an enormous blind date: I recognised some people from their profile pictures, but not others. Some were pregnant, some had babies and some were there without either a baby or a bump. I really felt for them; they were very brave.

Q: HOW MANY CYCLES OF IVF DO YOU THINK IT'S RIGHT TO HAVE?

At the first NHS clinic I went to, they told me that three was the maximum you should have. But at the ARGC, they told me that they learn more with every cycle. After four cycles, I used to trawl the internet looking for stories of women who'd been successful on their fifth cycle. Five was going to be our last cycle, but I'm sure that wouldn't be the right decision for everyone.

· · · · · · · · ·

So where does the controversy leave you, the patient who's simply hoping to get pregnant? If you have had repeated IVF failures, but with what your doctor says are good-quality embryos, you could read up to satisfy yourself that reproductive immunology is or is *not* the right choice for you.

To hear the arguments in favour, read about Dr Beer's theories at www.repro-med.net, or in his book, *Is Your Body Baby-Friendly?: Unexplained Infertility, Miscarriage and IVF Failure, Explained* (AJR Publishing). Or you can make an appointment at a clinic that practises reproductive immunology (such as the ARGC, Care Fertility, the Lister, Zita West Assisted Fertility).

Read up on the arguments against too. The RCOG guidelines are at www.rcog.org.uk/womens-health/clinical-guidance/immunological-testing-and-interventions-reproductive-failure and the HFEA advice is at www.hfea.gov.uk/fertility-treatment-options-reproductive-immunology.html.

Why I used
an egg donor

• • • • • • • • • • •

'Sixty-six-year-old to become Britain's oldest mother.'
'World's oldest mother gives birth to twins at 70.'
These are just two recent newspaper headlines on egg
donation. Whereas IVF has become normalised over the past
10 years, egg donation still makes headlines because it
provokes strong reactions, usually with an implication that
it's unnatural in some way. Val, whose story is below, had
treatment at the age of 45 and experienced this prejudice
first-hand, while on the examination table of a French gynaecologist. 'You should not be doing this, you should adopt
instead,' he told her.

It's true that egg donation shouldn't be taken lightly. 'You
do need to make a big emotional shift between IVF using
your own eggs, and IVF using donor eggs,' says fertility
coach, Anya Sizer. 'It's crucial that you don't [after IVF fail-
ure], just think that egg donation is simply your next option,'
she says. 'If you decide to go ahead, it's important – for you
and any possible child – that you explore all the ramifications

… The main fear that women I've spoken to have is, "Will the child feel like mine?" For some people, it will never feel enough. But for others, it's an incredible option, a chance of carrying a baby and giving birth to a child of their own.'

Marilyn Crawshaw, who has spent more than 25 years practising as a counsellor and doing research in this area and who contributes to parenting workshops for the Donor Conception Network, believes that counselling about the implications of donor conception is essential and might help you to avoid some of its pitfalls. 'Using a donor isn't something you can forget. It will be part of your family life and you need to feel ok about that.'

'You can never be 100 per cent sure about anything you're going to do, but counselling can help you to deal with any inevitable uncertainty.' Will you regret using donor eggs? How will you feel not having a child who's biologically related to you? What sort of personality will your child have? Will your child be curious about his or her origins?

The consensus is that the earlier the child knows that he or she was donor conceived, the better for him or her emotionally and so for you as a family. 'There's a whole life for you as parents and for your child to go through – all of you may view it differently at different times. Sharing your thoughts and experiences with others, especially other parents of donor conceived children, can help too, which is where the Donor Conception Network comes in.'

You also have to consider who's donating the eggs. In the UK, eggs come from altruistic anonymous donors or, increasingly, from friends or family; they can also come from egg-sharing schemes (see pages 172–3 for more information on all of these).

Finally, there's the question of anonymity. In the UK, children conceived since 2005 will be able to find out the identity of their biological parent and contact them, if they choose, at

18 (they are likely to get non-identifiable information much earlier). But in other countries where UK couples go for treatment, such as Spain, Greece and the Czech Republic, donors are anonymous, which means that the child has no legal right to trace their biological parent at any age, and matches are mostly made by doctors.

• • • • • • • • •

After 12 failed IVF treatments, Val, 45, a marketing manager from Sydney, Australia, travelled to Spain for treatment using donor eggs and sperm.

Crowded around the reception desk of our boutique hotel in Florence, my sister, Mum and I were all watching the hotel concierge intently. None of us could speak Italian, but we were hanging on his every word. He was on the phone to the clinic where I'd had a pregnancy blood test, asking them what the email of my results – in Italian – meant. Was I pregnant or not?

For what seemed like ages, the woman on the other end of the phone wouldn't tell him. Signora should fax the results on to her clinic in Spain, so they can tell her the result, she advised. But the concierge was persistent. He said – in Italian – 'Hypothetically speaking, if a person were to have these results, would they suggest she was pregnant?' And the woman replied, 'Yes'.

The whole lobby exploded into uproar. We started crying, as did the concierge, and we were hugging and kissing. Even the hotel manager joined in. He kept saying to Mum, 'You're going to be a nonna!' Some other guests came to check in, and they too got caught up in the excitement, hugging us as well. It's true what they say about the Italians – they do love babies! The hotel staff couldn't have been kinder or more caring.

We had travelled to Europe from Australia for me to have treatment with donor egg and sperm in Valencia, and we were taking in the sights of Italy and France too while we were there.

When I'd first set out to get pregnant, at the age of 41, neither egg donation nor going abroad was remotely what I'd imagined. I'd recently left a marriage of 15 years; my husband and I had always planned to have children but, due to his long illness, we'd put it off, year after year. Finally, wanting a child was too important to me to stay in my marriage. That left me at a loss, extremely sad not to have become a mother. But I was past the age of going to bars, and I couldn't imagine how to meet a new partner.

I began to think about using a sperm donor. I just hoped I hadn't left it too late. One day, driving Mum in the car, I said, 'You know I've always wanted a family? I'm thinking of using a donor.' She is quite conventional, and I wasn't sure how she'd react, but she said, 'What are you waiting for? Hurry up and get on with it.' She offered to support me in any way she could, emotionally, physically and financially.

At the clinic I chose in Sydney, the doctor recommended I go straight for IVF, due to my age. All my hormone tests were fine for a 41-year-old, and tests showed I didn't have any physical problems either. So it was time to select my sperm donor. There are Australian donors, but not many. I was offered 10 to 15 in total. It sounds a lot, but it isn't once you've taken ethnicity and age into account. In the end, there were two that sounded suitable. But then I found out that even if I picked one, I might not be able to use his sperm if another woman had done so recently because Australian donors are allowed a limit of 10 confirmed pregnancies.

My clinic had a relationship with a US clinic for importing sperm. They had plenty of donors, and although it was more expensive, I thought the choice was worth the money. So one night, I sat down at the kitchen table with my sister, a glass of red wine and my laptop, my mum doing chores in the background, and we logged on to the US donor clinic's database. Some of the donors provided a photo of themselves as children, and some also as adults, which I decided I wanted to see, to get a real sense of them. They described their own medical history, educational background, emotional traits and what they liked doing. And some wrote a blurb on why they were donating too. For some, it was because their wives had had a problem; others just wanted to help people. And one said he lived his life according to 'WWJD' – I looked it up, and found it meant, 'What would Jesus do?'

I was looking for a match that was close to my European background – I thought it was better for the child to look like me, as much as you can predict that sort of thing. It was quite funny, in the end, with Mum saying, 'You must go with him; he's the good-looking firefighter', as if he was a real suitor.

I eliminated all the young ones – the 19-year-olds – as being too weird to consider, especially after looking at their pictures. We must have looked through 400 donors, and I tried to pick those who sounded reasonably well-rounded. In the end, we all agreed on a guy who had a bit of Portuguese blood, an artistic, creative streak, a good academic record, a reasonably sound family health history and a sense of humour.

The clinic put me on a gruelling regime of stimulation drugs at very high doses. Some nights, I had to give myself six injections. It was quite stressful, holding down a job and rushing through the traffic to the clinic before work for scans. Sadly, the treatments failed, again and again. Most cycles, I produced up to eight eggs, with two to four of them not being viable, and had one or two embryos put back.

I'm quite an active person, and at first, I was doing lots of yoga, fast walking and outdoor workout programmes, trying to be healthy and in the best possible shape to conceive. But then I found out that too much hard exercise isn't always a good idea during IVF, so I cut back. I started to put on a lot of weight – mostly down to the drugs.

Usually, I'd get the call that the treatment had failed while I was at work, and I'd have to carry on as normal. I did tell one colleague, and he was comforting, but I couldn't let my emotions show, and that wore me down.

I didn't give myself a break between cycles to consider whether I should try again, but did IVF almost continuously for over three years. It took over my life; I missed overseas family weddings and all kinds of other social occasions. Historically, in my life and work, I've always been able to make things happen if I've tried hard enough, so even after five or six cycles, I was still reasonably optimistic it would work. But when it came to getting pregnant, I just couldn't make it happen. I kept mentally kicking myself for leaving it so late.

I felt like a battery chicken, totally pumped up with hormones. It definitely took its toll on my health, not just my weight. High cholesterol runs in my family, but mine went up so much that I had to see a cardiologist to test whether I was developing heart disease.

Eventually, after eight cycles, I decided to switch clinics. By this time, I'd read up about different approaches to treatment; my original clinic kept offering me the same protocol – the long one where you have to down-regulate – and I felt carrying on would have been like flogging a dead horse. At the new clinic, I switched to lower doses of the drugs, and tried the short antagonist protocol, where you go straight into stimulation, doing another injection to stop yourself ovulating too early.

My mum says I was like a zombie in the last year. And it's true – that time just went past in a blur of exhaustion and hormonal fug.

Then there was the cost. Every cycle cost $4000–5000 a go, with the sperm around $1000 to $1500 on top. With Medicare, the Australian public health system, I got around half of it back (although the law has since changed, so the refund is less). In the recovery room after an egg-collection procedure, I made friends with a woman who was around my age. We used to joke that we were having the world's most expensive babies – that once we'd had them, we'd have to live on bread and water for the rest of our lives.

I spent a lot on alternative treatments too. I did acupuncture twice a week for a number of cycles, as I'd read that might have an effect. But it was stressful trying to squeeze it into my lunch break, so I stopped. I also tried taking a disgusting, smelly concoction of Chinese herbs, which had a really nasty aftertaste. And I went to a natural fertility clinic, and was prescribed a whole list of specialist supplements. My salary soon disappeared.

By this point, I was 43 and running out of time. After 12 failed cycles, the clinic's advice was that IVF with my eggs most likely wouldn't work for me. In Australia, you have to provide your own egg donor, as donations must be a gift, not a financial transaction. For the last three or four IVF attempts, I'd felt that I should stop, but I couldn't face the reality of being childless. Going overseas for egg donation began to seem like a good option, if not my only one. And it was comforting that my mum and my sister said that if I did go, they would come with me.

I considered a clinic in South Africa, but I didn't think it was established enough. I also looked at California, but for the treatment alone it was 50,000 US dollars, with flights and accommodation to consider as well. Finally, I settled on Spain. There are some very well-established clinics there, and physically, the donors would be closer to my European heritage. We decided to turn the trip into a family holiday, staying in nice hotels and seeing the European sights.

The clinic I chose was professional and cutting-edge. It had been around for over 30 years, was reasonably large with a good reputation and a dedicated international department for overseas patients. The downside was the law on anonymity in Spain, which meant I wouldn't be able to pick either the sperm or the egg donor. It was hard to accept that I'd lose control – that I wouldn't know anything about my possible child's parents, and neither would he or she.

To request a donor, I simply had to fill in a form about my personal physical characteristics – I didn't even have a wish list. I was told the donors would be Spanish and, eventually, I was given their age and blood type. That's it, for ever. In Australia, at the age of 18, the child can find out his or her parents' identities, but in Spain, nothing – not even in a medical emergency.

The medical side of treatment with donor eggs and sperm was very simple – you don't need as many drugs if you're not producing the egg yourself. And having travelled together to Spain, I had my mum and sister there to support me when it came to the embryo transfer.

Because we were making our way across Europe while we waited for my pregnancy test, I was in Florence when I found out I was pregnant. And I was in Nice, 10 days later, when I started to bleed. I had severe cramps and began to panic. That night, I passed a huge clot and, overnight, my breasts stopped being tender. I had to wait until an ultrasound the next day to find out if I'd lost the baby, but I already knew. It was very traumatic, particularly as donor eggs have such a good success rate, of 60 to 75 per cent for the first attempt. I was so glad to be with Mum and my sister, not to be going through it on my own.

Then I had to decide if I was going to try again. My mum and sister were in favour, and I decided to go ahead. It wasn't practical for them to stay in Europe any longer than we'd planned, but I had to force them to go back to Australia. After they left, I did think: what on earth am I doing here, alone, on the wrong side of the world? It was one of my lowest points.

While I was waiting for the next cycle, I went to stay with a lovely and supportive friend in Paris. I had to have a scan, to make sure that I was ready for transfer, so my friend booked me in with a gynaecologist, who'd been recommended. He was in his late 50s, smartly dressed, and obviously well respected, as his waiting room was full.

As I lay there, my legs in the air (I felt as if I'd dropped my pants in every major city in southern Europe by then), he did a thorough examination that seemed to last for ages. Then came his bombshell. With his device still inserted in me, he said, 'I don't think you should go ahead with this treatment.' I said, 'Excuse me?' I thought I'd misunderstood him, as he had a very thick accent.

He went on, 'There's no physical problem, but you should not be doing this.' He said I should adopt. I tried to explain adoption as a single parent, at my age, was virtually impossible in my country. He said I should adopt from overseas, get a 'Benetton family'.

I couldn't believe what I was hearing, and couldn't explain myself as I'd started crying. He patted me on the knee, and said that in his country they didn't allow such things at my age. I was already emotionally wobbly, and it took me two or three days to get over what he had said. He had no right to make that moral judgment.

The following week, I had my second transfer in Spain. My visa had run out, which meant I couldn't stay in France, and had to travel to London. It was there, on my own, that I booked in for a blood test and discovered I was pregnant again. I was happy, but cautious. A scan at five weeks showed two sacs – it looked as if both embryos might have taken.

The first cycle, I'd arranged to fly home when I was six weeks pregnant, but then I'd had the miscarriage. I was worried it was too early to make such a long-haul flight, but I was desperate to get home. On the day of my flight, I started bleeding. I was terrified – could this really be happening again? A friend found me a clinic where I could have an emergency scan, and as I lay on the examination table, I dreaded what I was going to see. Then I saw a sac, and the doctor said, 'There's the heartbeat'. I cried with relief; it was so incredible. The bleeding had probably come from the other embryo, which hadn't made it.

I have never been so pleased to be home with my family, who were so delighted for me. The pregnancy was quite gruelling physically for the first five months, as I had severe morning sickness and fatigue. But it got easier after that, and I started enjoying it.

I'd thought that due to my age, the birth would be harder, but I stayed calm and there were no complications at all. I was a little bit in awe when I first saw Freddie – especially as I'd expected him to be a girl! Straight away, it felt very natural to have him, and feed him, and it's been like that ever since.

Even though Freddie's not my biological child, he feels like mine – he even looks a bit like me, with lots of dark hair. He's now six weeks old and I can't imagine not being a mum, even though I didn't think it would ever happen.

I would have given up sooner if it wasn't for the support of my family. My intention, all my life, was to have a child; it just didn't work out before.

Q: HOW DID YOU KNOW THAT USING DONOR EGGS WAS RIGHT FOR YOU?

In my extended family, there's one adopted person and one who has never known her father. It was clear to me from them that DNA doesn't necessarily make a parent.

After several failed IVF attempts, I started to explore foster care and adoption in Australia, only to discover how much of a difficult, bureaucratic and lengthy process it was going to be, and there was no guarantee of success. Simply put, being single and older made it extremely unlikely that I'd end up being able to adopt.

I originally discounted donor eggs because of the cost, and the fact that there are no clinics that offer them in Australia. You have to find your own donor. Early on, my sister who, at 37, was younger than me offered to be an egg donor. It was quite a gift. I didn't want her to do it at first – she has polycystic ovaries and other health issues, so I knew it would be hard for her, and I felt guilty about putting her through the gruelling process of IVF. After I'd had eight IVF attempts, I accepted her offer and she did an egg-donation cycle. She produced one viable embryo, but it didn't take.

Although being biologically related to my child started out being extremely important to me, once I realised I was willing to adopt, I also realised I'd already accepted having a non-biological child. The fact I would be carrying, nurturing and then giving birth to the child myself made me feel even more positive about using an egg donor.

Q: DID YOU THINK THROUGH THE FUTURE IMPLICATIONS OF DONOR ANONYMITY?

It took me months to consider emotionally, research and finally accept egg donation as an option for me. Because both the sperm donor and egg donor were anonymous in my case, I had a lot to think about. The easiest way for me to handle it was to think that if I adopted a child, I would more than likely know nothing about the birth parents. Freddie may feel different at some point in his life, and I will have to cross that bridge when we come to it.

Q: HAVE YOU DECIDED WHAT YOU WILL TELL FREDDIE AS HE IS GROWING UP?

That's probably one of the most difficult decisions. While I have done some research on this, I am undecided as to when is the right time. There is no doubt that Freddie will know how he came about and the journey I took to have him. I intend on being as open and honest as possible. I personally believe that as soon as a child is mature enough and emotionally equipped to process this kind of information, that's the time to tell them. I definitely don't want to leave it until Freddie is an adult.

Q: WHAT WOULD YOU TELL YOUR 41-YEAR-OLD SELF, WHO WAS JUST STARTING TREATMENT?

Goodness, I was naive when I started. I would tell her to do more research – I had no idea how low my chance was of succeeding, statistically. By the time I was 43, it was down to less than 5 per cent.

I'd also tell her to be very clear at what point she'd stop, and explore other options. Initially, I decided to do three cycles. But then I found it very hard to stop, to give up my dream of a family. I also should have thought about trying a donor-egg cycle earlier on. But the clinics in Australia aren't allowed to be seen to be actively co-operating with an overseas service, so it wasn't until later on that I discovered it was an option.

Q: WAS IT HARD TO BE AWAY FROM HOME?

It was fine at first, when Mum and my sister were with me. There was the language barrier, of course, which made it hard to arrange all the scans, drugs and blood tests I needed in different countries. But after they went home, when I'd been in Europe for three months, I was really homesick. I knew that, even if something went wrong with the pregnancy, I could deal with it better surrounded by family.

Q: HOW HAVE PEOPLE REACTED TO FREDDIE BEING AN EGG-DONOR CHILD?

My family and friends are really enjoying Freddie. They joke that I had a four-year pregnancy! The story of how he was conceived went around the hospital like wildfire, and lots of the nurses said nice things. Quite a few people have told me they really admire what I did, and others have got in touch because they want to go overseas for egg donation too. I suppose anyone disapproving doesn't say anything. But I don't care one bit. Freddie is what matters.

• • • • • • • • •

In the UK, eggs come from three sources. Firstly, friends and family donate (known donors which, says Marilyn Crawshaw, needs to be carefully managed). Secondly, some women choose to donate anonymously as a selfless act, sometimes because they, or someone they know, have had fertility problems (altruistic donors); the organisation Altrui (altrui.org.uk) campaigns to encourage more women to come forward as donors. Finally, some clinics offer free or cut-price IVF in return for women giving away half the eggs collected (egg sharing). Views on this last option vary. Anya Sizer describes it as 'an incredible option, where a woman who's having IVF treatment does something altruistic for another woman', while Crawshaw says it is often driven by financial motives: 'would the donor be giving away half of her eggs if she could afford IVF?' she asks.

Egg-donation counselling should be offered at your clinic (find a counsellor at bica.net). Now, any children conceived in the UK will be able to trace their biological parents when aged 18 (for more information, see the Donor Conception Network, dcnetwork.org). The DCN website is a useful source of real-life stories too.

There is still a shortage of egg donors in the UK, which is why so many couples choose to go abroad. More information is available from the National Gamete Donation Trust at ngdt. co.uk.

However, the good news is that the success rate with donated eggs is high because it depends on egg quality, and donors in the UK have to be under 36, as well as healthy.

My experience
of surrogacy

• • • • • • • • • • • • •

lthough surrogacy might have got an exclusive, expensive reputation, with Nicole Kidman and Sarah Jessica Parker admitting to having needed a 'gestational carrier', the reality is that it's for normal people too. 'The reason people choose surrogacy isn't that they're too scared or lazy to carry a child, or worried about losing their figure,' says Linda Nelson, chairperson of Childlessness Overcome Through Surrogacy (COTS), a long-established surrogacy agency. 'It's because they have no choice. Mostly, they've been through horrendous fertility or medical problems. Surrogacy isn't anyone's first option.'

But how do you know if surrogacy is for you? 'As surrogacy is becoming more acceptable, it's also becoming more popular,' says Linda. 'But that doesn't mean it's right for you. One test is: if you couldn't say to friends and family that you're having a surrogate baby, it's probably not.'

It's in no way easy, either. 'There are generally more couples wanting surrogates than there are surrogates,' says

Linda, 'particularly for "straight" surrogates, where the surrogate uses her own eggs.'

And the legal situation is tricky too. 'The law tries to protect the woman who gives birth and her husband,' says Natalie Gamble, a solicitor who specialises in fertility law. 'In surrogacy cases, it means you end up with the wrong people being the parents. The surrogate will always be the mother and, if she's married, her husband will be the father.

'There's then a legal process that the parents have to go through after the birth in order to reassign parenthood and get a birth certificate which names them as the parents. It can be straightforward, provided you meet all the criteria. In most UK cases, the intended parents can do it themselves.'

Surrogacy isn't allowed to be a commercial agreement in the UK – the surrogate can only be paid expenses – and the actual surrogacy agreement isn't legally binding. That means that it's done on trust. 'It isn't a business arrangement,' says Linda. 'It's something one person wants to do to help another.'

The implications of this are that the surrogate – the legal mother – could, in theory, decide not to give the baby to the intended parents and the courts could agree. That's what happened in a recent court case about Baby T. 'Actually, surrogacy arrangements going wrong is incredibly rare,' says Gamble. 'But intended parents, understandably, worry about it a great deal. This was the very first case reported in the UK of a surrogate being allowed to keep the baby. There was one previous case of a dispute, where the intended parents won care. In any case like this, the court makes its decision depending on what it thinks is in the child's best interests.'

Then there's the issue of money. Surrogacy might not be commercial, but the courts accept payments for expenses of up to around £12,000 as being reasonable. And you also have to pay the cost of IVF, if you're able to use your own eggs, in a host surrogacy arrangement. That could make it unaffordable for a lot of couples unless a member of the family or a friend volunteers to be their surrogate. 'From a surrogate's point of view,' says Linda, 'twelve thousand pounds isn't a lot of money. It can be months trying to get pregnant, then nine months of pregnancy. The amount isn't unreasonable when you consider that it could take up to two years and, as safe as childbirth is now, the surrogate is still putting her life and health on the line.'

The situation is much more confusing with surrogacy abroad, mainly because UK law still applies, wherever in the world the baby is born. 'The law concerning the child's nationality and getting him or her back into the UK is complicated,' says Gamble. 'And when you make an application to the court to become legal parents here, your situation will be looked at very carefully, particularly if you have entered into a commercial surrogacy arrangement abroad. Before approving you as the parents, the court will look into all the details very carefully to make sure that there has been no exploitation, the order is in your child's best interests and that you did everything properly in the foreign country.'

Having said all of this, most of the time, surrogacy is relatively problem-free. 'Surrogacy won't have been your first option,' says Linda, 'but when it works, it's brillliant. Ideally, the surrogacy arrangement will end up with both families being friends for life.'

• • • • • • • •

After a labour that almost killed her, Tanja, 42, an operations manager from Glasgow, was told she could never carry a baby again.

Douglas and I were in the playground at our boys' school when we got an unexpected call to say that we'd been chosen by a surrogate. She wanted to carry our baby. I heard Douglas say, 'Hello Jay', when he answered his mobile, so I knew it was the agency. Then he burst into tears and I could see, straight away, that it was good news. We'd only posted our request a few days before, so we weren't expecting to hear for ages. I thought: oh my goodness, we might actually have another baby. Then I cried too.

Nikki, our potential surrogate, had chosen us as soon as she read our story. In our request, we had explained that our baby, Lola, had died a few months before because my uterus ruptured during her birth. We'd written that if Douglas, myself and our sons, Kian, who was six, and Josh, three, were going to heal as a family, we needed to have another baby.

The story first began after Josh was born. In fact, it was then that we decided not to have a third child. But if we'd been serious about not wanting one, I suppose we'd have been serious about using contraception too. Douglas did go on a waiting list for a vasectomy but, in the meantime, we didn't take any precautions, apart from trying to avoid my fertile time. We were playing Russian roulette, really, due to my irregular cycle, and I fell pregnant accidentally early in 2008. A week later we received a letter from the clinic booking Douglas in for his vasectomy. Just a little too late!

Sadly, at 12 and a half weeks, a scan showed the baby had died. The miscarriage was caused by a virus that the whole family had caught – slapped cheek syndrome (parvovirus B19), so called because the main symptom is a bright red facial rash.

I had to go into hospital to be induced and to deliver the foetus, which was as awful and sad as it sounds. I was horrified when my waters broke – I hadn't expected that to happen – and burst into tears. Twenty minutes later, I passed the pregnancy. Although I knew it was only a foetus, I couldn't help but think of it as a baby.

I was upset for months after that, and because we didn't want our last memory of pregnancy to be so awful, Douglas and I decided to try for another child. I began using ovulation kits and, six months later, I was pregnant. At 20 weeks, we found out the baby was a girl. I thought ours would be a perfect family: two boys and a girl, each three years apart.

The pregnancy was uneventful, although I was in a lot of discomfort towards the end, as the baby was lying horizontally, which they call transverse. At 37 weeks, the doctor decided to turn her to the head-down position, which he did with his hands on my tummy, and she moved very easily. But by the time I got home a few hours later, she was transverse again. Then at 38 weeks, she was head down.

At 39 weeks, the doctor thought she was transverse again, and said that the best course of action would be to turn her again, then induce my labour. He said, 'We don't want to give you a C-section, do we?' It was such a flippant remark, but it's one that's stayed with me ever since. The pros and cons of a C-section weren't discussed at that point, although I suppose because I'd already had two normal deliveries, there wasn't much reason for the doctor to recommend one. Douglas wasn't with me that day, and I can't help thinking he would have been another ear, and may have questioned the doctor a bit more than I did. There had been some talk of a C-section a few weeks before though and, at the time, Douglas and I had decided it probably wasn't a good idea for practical reasons, with two children and no family around to provide support.

All the same, I was terrified of another labour, especially since I was told that the baby was big. Kian had been induced, as my waters had broken without contractions, and he'd passed meconium, so the doctor wanted to get him out quickly. I'd had an epidural because induced contractions are very painful. With Josh there wasn't time for an epidural. I'd tried gas and air, but it made me sick, so I had only diamorphine, which did nothing.

I didn't know if I'd be able to push a big baby out, and I was dreading the pain, even with an epidural. I wanted the easy option of a C-section, but then thought I was being wimpy. I look back now and think: I wish I'd had that C-section.

The labour started out on track. I had the pessary to open up my cervix, then my waters broke and I was put on an oxytocin drip to stimulate my contractions, and given an epidural. Even with the pain relief I could feel the contractions; they're pretty bloody strong when you're induced. Once I was fully dilated, five hours later, I was told to push. I pushed for around 40 minutes, but nothing happened. With hindsight, this being my third baby, Lola should have come out pretty easily, probably in less than 20 minutes. The midwife said she could see the head in the birth canal, so there was no reason to think she wasn't going to come out.

Suddenly, Lola's heart rate dipped, and my contractions stopped. The midwife said, very calmly, 'I think the baby is a bit stressed. I'm going to call the doctor.' The registrar came into the room, and from then on, it was pandemonium. The quickest way to get a baby out at that point is with forceps, but when the registrar went to do a forceps delivery, Lola wasn't in the birth canal any more. No one knew at that stage, but my uterus had ruptured, and Lola had fallen into my abdominal cavity.

I was rushed to theatre for a crash C-section and knocked out. The registrar said that when she opened me up, she'd never seen anything like it before. There was a split the shape of an inverted 'Y' down the back of my uterus, and it had come away from my cervix. Lola didn't have a heartbeat.

There was one team of doctors working on me, stitching me back together, and one on Lola. They did manage to resuscitate her about 30 minutes later; there was a very very faint heartbeat, but it wasn't sustainable.

I was in surgery for three hours. I was told later that, for the first hour and a half, the surgeons were trying to save my life. I lost four litres of blood. Doctors came from other parts of the hospital to assist with the surgery as the damage was so extreme. None of them had ever seen a uterine rupture before – it's very rare.

Douglas was in the room next door with absolutely no idea of what was happening. Finally, the consultant paediatrician came out and told him that the baby was in a critical condition, that she wasn't going to make it, and asked if he'd like to see her. They brought Lola to him; at the time, she had a faint heartbeat, but she died in his arms. Douglas was left holding his dead daughter, wondering what on earth he was going to say to me. He called my mum and my sister in New Zealand and broke down, saying, 'How am I going to tell Tanja?'

When I woke up, four and a half hours later, the first person I saw was the paediatrician. And the first words I said were, 'Is the baby ok?' He said, 'I'll just get your husband', and I just knew. I don't remember Douglas' exact words, but I started screaming, saying, 'It's not true. It's not true.'

The rest of that time is a blur. I was still completely out of it, and on a morphine drip, but, apparently, I asked to see

Lola. I couldn't hold her because of the surgery, but they laid her next to me in the bed. She was all wrapped up, and I tried to unwrap her. Douglas tried to stop me, but I said, 'No. I want to see her from top to toe.' She was perfect, not a mark on her. She looked just like she was sleeping, as if you could wake her up.

It wasn't until the next day that the doctors told Douglas how close he'd come to losing me too, that the surgery had been so major. In hospital, I was kept in a room on the delivery ward, so I wouldn't be surrounded by other mums and babies, I suppose. I had to stay in for a week to be monitored. I had a catheter because of the trauma to my bladder, and another blood transfusion two days later.

The nurses brought Lola to me whenever I wanted to see her, but after a few days it became quite frightening, as she'd changed so much in appearance, and that wasn't how I wanted to remember her.

On the ward, there were women giving birth all around me; I turned up the TV so I couldn't hear them. The midwives were fantastic, very compassionate and always there when I needed to talk and cry. One, in particular, took over all the funeral arrangements and looked after both my husband and me.

I did cry in hospital, but not as much as I did later on – I think because I was still in shock. All week, my brain was constantly churning, and I was thinking: what if I'd had a C-section? Douglas kept saying to me, 'You've got to stop thinking that. It's not as if you had a choice.' But if I'd said I wanted one, would the doctor have done it?

I kept reliving those last moments of labour, again and again. I felt very angry towards the midwife. There had been a change of shift during the evening, and I hadn't bonded with the new midwife. I'd found her very clinical. Had she been complacent because it was my third child, I wondered?

She kept telling me to push and nothing was happening – because my uterus had ruptured. At the time, I wanted to say, 'I am fucking pushing'.

You're so out of it during labour; you forget everything you've been taught in classes or read in books. I kept thinking: why didn't she ask me how I was, or what sensations I was feeling? She didn't *do* anything wrong – she was following all the guidelines for an induced labour (that the drugs should only induce a maximum of four heavy contractions every 10 minutes); but if she'd been more in touch with me, would she have known my uterus had ruptured? (In fact, as a result of what happened to me, they've since changed the induced-labour guidelines for someone who's had previous deliveries to a maximum of three contractions every 10 minutes.) But uterine rupture is so rare – one in 15,000 if you've never had a Caesarean or uterine surgery – should she really have been aware of the possibility?

When the consultant came to talk to me in hospital, she explained that Lola's head probably wasn't in the right position when I was pushing. So although she looked as if she was going to come down the birth canal, she was stuck. And all the pressure from the induced contractions built up behind her. Eventually something had to give, and it was my uterus. I kept thinking: so if I was pushing and nothing was happening, why did the midwife wait until Lola's heartbeat dipped?

Kian, my older son, came to hospital to see me, but Josh, at three, was too little. Kian held Lola and said goodbye to her. He was in tears too. Both the boys had been so excited about having a little sister. The day of the birth, we'd told them, 'Mummy will be home soon with the baby', then suddenly we had to tell them a new story.

After a week, I was allowed home. I was fearful of seeing the empty nursery, and my sons' reactions, especially the three-year-old's. He kept going into Lola's room and looking in her cot, saying, 'Where's the baby, Mummy? Is the baby not coming home?' Kian didn't want to talk about Lola; he was like a little scared rabbit.

I was a zombie, not knowing what to do with myself. I felt as if I should have been at home nursing my baby, but I just kept walking round in circles. When the health visitor came to see me, it was awful as I kept thinking, 'Why are you here? You should be here because I have a new baby and I don't.'

All I thought about was Lola, from the moment I woke to when I went to sleep. I was having a lot of nightmares, due to the trauma and grief. I'd sit in Lola's room, in the rocking chair I'd put in there for breastfeeding. We'd bought a cot bumper and duvet cover to match the new pink wallpaper, and there were drawers full of pretty clothes. Kian had chosen her coming-home outfit, and it was still laid out, completely untouched. It was a very peaceful, beautiful room, the last in the house to get the sun.

We couldn't face Christmas or New Year, so two weeks after I got out of hospital, we went to Florida for a month. We just wanted to escape, hoping that by the time we came back, everybody would know and we wouldn't need to keep explaining. Douglas had already had to do enough ringing around to tell people.

Lots of people wrote to us. It was a comfort to know that so many people were thinking of us, but at the same time, it felt so wrong to have a house full of sympathy cards instead of congratulation ones.

When the initial shock had worn off, after a couple of months, Douglas and I started to talk about trying for a baby. I had been very strongly advised by my consultant in hospital not to get pregnant. But we knew that the only way we could heal would be to have another baby. In fact, Douglas had already started to look into adoption and surrogacy, although he didn't tell me at the time because I wasn't ready.

When we did talk, I said I wanted to adopt because I wanted a little girl, and I couldn't guarantee that if we went down the surrogacy route. And I told Douglas that if we were going to do surrogacy, I wanted a 'straight' surrogate, that is someone who uses her own eggs. I couldn't bear any more gynaecological prodding and poking.

Douglas contacted the surrogacy agency COTS (Childlessness Overcome Through Surrogacy), but discovered that because straight surrogates were in short supply the list for them was closed. So we decided then that we would try for IVF and a 'gestational' surrogate who would carry our biological baby.

Douglas did all the groundwork. I was so caught up in my grief that I couldn't think. My children were the only reason I got out of bed. I still couldn't go anywhere near the school playground. I couldn't believe I wasn't there with my pram and everybody fussing around the baby. I felt like a leper, as if people were looking at me, not knowing what to say because my self-esteem and confidence had been knocked so much.

When we first went to the IVF clinic, I did a blood test for the hormone AMH, to find out how fertile I was. Luckily, the results were good for my age as, at 42, the odds for IVF weren't stacked in my favour. But we looked at it from the point of view that IVF is for people with fertility problems, and we didn't have any. We were given a 22 per cent chance of the treatment working – or 29 per cent if we opted for assisted hatching, where the embryologist makes a hole in the embryo's outer layer to help it to expand.

Because fertility decreases so fast after the age of 40, the clinic doctor advised us to do an IVF cycle straight away, then to freeze the embryos. I went through a cycle with absolutely no side effects whatsoever and produced eight eggs. Six fertilised with Douglas' sperm, and they were all frozen.

Meanwhile, we started the process to look for a surrogate. First, you pay a fee to join the surrogacy agency, and you supply a description of yourself, your partner and your family, and why you need help. If you're chosen, you pay the surrogate's expenses, for travel and childcare and so on, around £10,000. It isn't supposed to be a commercial arrangement.

I called Nikki as soon as we got home from the parents' evening. It was nerve-wracking. We didn't talk about surrogacy at all; we just talked about ourselves and our backgrounds and got to know each other a little. It didn't seem real to be talking to the woman who potentially was going to carry our baby for us, and give us that incredible gift of new life. She told me she was 28, and had four girls: a six-year-old, a three-year-old and seven-month-old twins. She'd never been a surrogate before.

We arranged to meet – just the two of us – to see if we clicked. And we got on really well. Douglas was desperate to meet Nikki too, and a couple of weeks later, both familes went to a soft-play area, so the kids could have fun while we talked. Douglas and I really liked Nikki and her husband too. She's a genuinely lovely person and a really good mum – a very level-headed, switched-on woman. I could tell that being a surrogate was something she truly wanted to do, that she wasn't in it for the money. And I knew she'd look after our baby.

The agency drew up an agreement, and we all signed it. It's not legally binding, but the idea is that all the details – payments, expenses, the birth – are set out clearly before you begin. Once it's signed, you're left to get on with things.

By law, you have to wait six months – a quarantine period – before you can transfer human cells into another person's body. That was very frustrating, as we just wanted to get on with getting pregnant. So our clinic wrote to the HFEA stating our case, including my age, and they waived the six months. Douglas and I had already had our medical checkups so, once Nikki had had hers, we were ready to go.

On the day that Nikki's cycle was right for the embryo transfer, I had had to travel to Sydney. So Douglas got dressed up in scrubs and went into theatre with her. He said it was very weird, being there with a woman who wasn't his wife at such an intimate moment. It was 10 a.m. in the UK and 10 p.m. where I was, and Nikki and Douglas sent me photos of the doctors and of Nikki lying on the bed, to make me feel part of it. It was pretty surreal.

Ten days later, on the day she could do a pregnancy test, Nikki invited us for dinner, so we could be there. And the test was positive. Douglas cried, but I didn't. In the car on the way home, he said I seemed detached, but it was because I was still trying to get my head around the fact that another woman would be giving birth to our baby. Men can often be removed from pregnancy because they don't carry the baby. And my counsellor says that even if I was carrying the baby myself, I might have been detached, as a protection mechanism after the trauma I'd been through.

At the 18-week scan, we found out that we were having a boy. That was when we finally started talking about names, too. I was so happy he was healthy, but I also had to work through the fact that I'd lost my dream of ever having a daughter. I'm not going to lie and say I wasn't disappointed, but I did know this baby would be absolutely loved.

I joined an online forum for women who've had uterine rupture, and started exchanging emails with someone who had the same experience a year before Lola died, and lost her son. Her surrogate was pregnant at the same time as mine. It was good to speak to someone who'd been through the same as me, and to realise that what I was feeling was normal.

It was horrendous leading up to the birth. People kept asking me if I was excited, but that was the emotion that was furthest from the way I was feeling, which was more like terror. I thought the birth would drag all my emotions over Lola back up, but in the end none of that happened.

Of course, like all babies, this one came when he wasn't expected – we were out having an early celebration for our tenth wedding anniversary. So Douglas and I arrived at the hospital straight from the restaurant, me in dress and heels. Although Nikki lives 45 minutes away from us, our consultant came from home to Nikki's hospital to oversee things. I think she wanted and needed to see this baby born safely, too.

I hadn't planned to be in the room during the birth. But I was there when the midwife said that things would be happening soon, and Nikki grabbed my hand, and asked me to stay with her. Forty minutes later, the baby was delivered safely. And I caught him as he came out, screaming, which was lovely to hear.

It was really emotional – Douglas and I both sobbed and sobbed. And Douglas cut the cord. Then we sat and held him, which was incredible. The relief was overwhelming that we had a living, screaming baby. We decided to call him Cory Nicholas as Cory means 'God's peace' and Nicholas after Nikki.

Nikki had the second cuddle after us. She told me later that her first thought after the birth was, 'That's not my baby'.

Nikki went home after four hours, leaving Douglas and I to look after Cory. I had been nervous about whether I'd bond with him, but there was no problem with that at all.

Four weeks later, and I love him to pieces. He has brought a lot of peace and happiness to our family. Douglas says he's put our family back together. Last week, my elder son said: 'I'll never forget Lola, but if she had come home, we wouldn't have needed to have had Cory.' And the younger one can't stop holding and kissing him, singing songs and helping with nappies.

We've seen Nikki a couple of times since. She said she had just one day of feeling down after the birth. We'll tell Cory that she did an amazing thing for us by carrying him. And we'll stay in touch with Nikki, hopefully see her a few times a year. We gave her a bracelet charm with the letter C and one with Cory's birthstone, and a huge bunch of flowers saying 'thank you to my tummy mummy, from Cory'. And I'm going to get his footprints done in pottery for her, too.

I've been feeling a mixture of emotions, but much more happiness than sadness. I do think about Lola. She will never be forgotten, and the pain surrounding her loss will be there forever. And I feel sad that I couldn't carry Cory and never will carry a baby again. But that doesn't make any difference to the way I feel about him.

I'm up a lot at night, of course, but I don't resent one minute of it. I would be happy if I was up every single hour, every night. I love that people stop me to look in the pram. We've had so many cards and presents for him, even from people I hardly know, that the living room is completely full. Douglas says it's nice to see me smiling again. A friend summed it up when she said, 'when Cory arrived, everyone who knew what had happened breathed a sigh of relief'.

Q: IN WHAT WAYS WAS HAVING A SURROGATE CARRIER DIFFERENT FROM WHAT YOU EXPECTED?

I can't say I had any expectations about how I would feel. It is such a different experience, I'd say it's impossible to predict your own personal reaction. The only insight we had came from speaking to other parents going through a surrogacy arrangement and from our own surrogate. Although it was her first time, Nikki read up a lot and she shared her knowledge with us. We talked to other parents and surrogates on the COTS forum, discussing feelings and problems and asking questions, which was very useful.

Q: HOW DID YOU FEEL ABOUT HAVING A SURROGATE CARRIER?

I think I found it harder than Douglas, as it was the first time that I was physically detached from a pregnancy – whereas the man always is. At times, I did have some feelings of jealousy and even a little resentment at the fact she could so easily carry our baby. I thought: why can't that be me?

I would say both Douglas and I felt somewhat distanced from the whole process. Douglas, for example, was too nervous to ask Nikki if he could feel her tummy. It didn't seem as exciting as carrying the baby ourselves and we didn't feel the same emotions as when I was pregnant. I think a lot of that was also fear though – we were scared to get too attached in case something happened to the baby again.

Q: HOW DID YOU EXPLAIN ABOUT THE BABY TO YOUR BOYS?

Our boys were very excited when we told them. Kian, who's now seven, said it made him feel 'a lot happier'. Our younger son Josh went straight to nursery the next day and said, 'I'm having another baby but it's not in my mummy's tummy' – so that was that out of the bag!

Kian was very interested to know how it had all happened, so Douglas had an interesting conversation with him about doctors making things in petri dishes. I asked him if he had had any awkward questions at school about why the baby wasn't in his mummy's tummy and he just said, 'That's not important, Mummy'. Josh often asked when we were planning to visit our surrogate and, 'Are we getting the baby today?'

I've been really surprised at how they both took it in their stride.

Q: WERE YOU LOOKING FORWARD TO THE BIRTH?

To be honest, I was terrified. We decided that only Douglas would be present in the delivery room with Nikki. I was worried about all the emotions it might bring up around the loss of Lola. I didn't think I would be of any help in keeping Nikki calm and relaxed. I think Douglas also felt somewhat anxious about the emotions that labour might stir up again, but we were both prepared for that, at least. And I knew I'd feel relief and joy when the baby was finally in our arms.

• • • • • • • • •

The established surrogacy agencies (COTS at surrogacy.org. uk, Surrogacy UK at surrogacyuk.org and A Little Wish at a-little-wish.co.uk) are an ideal place to start, as they have experience dealing with all the usual problems that can arise. The most common, according to COTS chairperson Linda Nelson, is a lack of contact between the surrogate and parents, or sometimes even too much contact. 'The surrogate shouldn't feel neglected, but she shouldn't feel overwhelmed either,' says Linda. Deciding these kinds of details in advance, and getting them down in an agreement, means everyone has something in writing that they can look back on, even if it's not legally binding. Also, agencies interview surrogates in advance to make sure that surrogacy is right for them, and they are right for surrogacy.

Parents and surrogates can also connect via websites. But, according to Linda, 'The problem with some websites is, if something goes wrong, you're on your own'. Agencies will help you with the legal side and guide you through the process of applying for a parental order, which is what you need to become the child's legal parents. Solicitors Natalie Gamble Associates have lots of clear information on the legal side on their website too (www.nataliegambleassociates. com). Do your research before you start, and don't rush into surrogacy abroad without checking out the law, as it could save you time, money and a lot of heartache in the future. There aren't many books written about surrogacy in the UK; the US books are good for real stories, but not for the how-tos. There's *Surrogacy and Embryo, Sperm & Egg Donation: What Were You Thinking?* by Theresa M. Erickson (iUniverse.com), a guide to all the issues that might come up, and *Surrogacy Was the Way: Twenty Intended Mothers Tell Their Stories* by Zara Griswold (Nightengale Press).

I got pregnant naturally after IVF

• • • • • • • • • • • •

The first time I did IVF, I researched obsessively online and, every time I read a study or about a treatment, I'd change my behaviour. I gave up alcohol and coffee, switched to organic food, cleaning products and shampoo, had my mercury-containing fillings removed, took handfuls of supplements, had acupuncture, cranial osteopathy (great for my neck), reflexology (which felt just like a foot massage) and hypnotherapy (which I hated). As one friend, Nicola, who was also having IVF at the same time said, 'You never know if the one thing you didn't try is the one that would have worked.' She was the person who introduced me to wearing Primark's orange knickers during treatment, as orange is, supposedly, the colour of fertility. Obsessive, moi?

For my second and third cycles, I tried to be more balanced. I stopped drinking, but I ate non-organic food and used my usual shampoo. I had the one treatment that always made me feel better: acupuncture with Emma Cannon, an acupuncturist specialising in pregnancy and fertility. I saw nutritionist Marilyn Glenville for advice on supplements for ageing eggs (she added selenium, vitamin D, omega 3 oils and vitamin C to my fertility multivitamin) and I spent a luxurious week doing a 'detox' at the Original MAYR clinic in Austria, who say that their programme prepares you to get pregnant.

Looking back, I can see I was still pretty obsessed. But I'm not the only one. As is the case with almost all the women I interviewed for this book, fertility took over my life.

Another friend, Helen, worked out that she spent over £2500 on acupuncture, herbs, supplements, hypnotherapy and seeing nutritionists while trying to conceive her son Harry.

Professor Bill Ledger thinks this is one of the dangers of alternative therapies. 'They shouldn't be costing you a lot of money, especially if your funds are limited,' he says. 'If you're spending thousands of pounds on them, I'd advise it might be better to keep the money, and spend it on another cycle of IVF.' That's because, he says, there isn't much scientific proof that most natural therapies can increase your chances of pregnancy. 'The first thing I say to patients is, make sure any therapies are harmless,' he says. 'Then, there are certain things that we know are physical causes of infertility, such as when the man has no sperm, or the woman has blocked Fallopian tubes. These are not going to be fixed by anything other than a clinical approach. But for quite a lot of people who have unexplained infertility, or a mild male problem, or maybe the woman doesn't ovulate every month, complementary therapies may be helpful as they may improve your sense of wellbeing, and that can affect the body.'

Don't be afraid to ask therapists for evidence that their therapies can help. Nutrition and acupuncture, for example, are two that have some positive studies backing them up (although there are negative ones too).

'Finally,' says Professor Ledger, 'you shouldn't spend years having complementary therapies without getting a medical diagnosis, especially if the woman is 30 or over. Otherwise, by the time you do get a diagnosis, your age may have become a factor.' Fertility expert and acupuncturist Zita West agrees: 'Complementary therapies need to work within a medical plan and time frame, so that no valuable fertility time is wasted,' she says. So if your practitioner is advising you to hold off from having medical treatment to wait for their therapy to 'work', make sure your doctor knows about it.

Acupuncturist Emma Cannon says, 'Complementary therapies address the whole person and also, particularly, the emotions which are often overlooked in medical treatment.' And practitioners have time to talk, which doctors don't. 'In Chinese medicine, your personal experience of your health is central to your diagnosis and treatment, and that can be immensely empowering to the patient,' she says.

• • • • • • • • •

Kate, 38, from Wiltshire, had three cycles of IUI and three rounds of IVF then got pregnant naturally.

My periods stopped at 15, which doctors put down to exam stress and playing a lot of sport – netball, athletics and swimming. At university, I couldn't understand it when, in my second year, despite still playing a lot of sport, I went from a size 10 to a size 16. My hair started falling out and my energy dropped dramatically, so that I struggled to get to lectures, then, as my symptoms worsened, to do anything but sleep all day and night.

All classic signs of a severely underactive thyroid, I found out when I was finally diagnosed. But mine was so underactive that I was told I could have been six months away from dying.

On top of that scary diagnosis, you know how sometimes doctors can handle situations completely the wrong way? Well, this was one of those times. My GP was looking over my notes and said, 'And you've got polycystic ovaries too. You do realise that will mean you'll never have children?' I came out of her surgery in a trance, shocked. But it wasn't until I got back to my digs and called my parents that I started crying. Even though I didn't want children right that minute, I knew I wanted them at some point. Mummy tried to be positive, saying, 'First we'll work on getting your thyroid better, then your periods will start again.'

I was only 24 when I met Peter, but we were pretty serious from the word go. My thyroid was under control with medication, but my periods hadn't come back – I'd had just one in the previous two years – and I felt I had to be up front about that. So a few months after we met, I told him that I couldn't get pregnant, so if he wanted children, he really should go and find somebody who could. Peter told me not to be so bloody stupid; he said he knew he wanted to marry me and that, somehow, we would have our family. But I've had times – a lot of them – when I've thought it would never happen; moments of complete darkness, of despair. During the six years we were trying, while four doctors gave up on us and referred us to another clinic, Peter never gave up.

When we first got married, we hoped for the best, that it would just take a little longer than normal to get pregnant. My GP told me to try for six months, though I still wasn't having periods. Then he referred me to our local hospital for fertility tests: blood tests, ultrasound scans, and a laparoscopy to look inside me and check my tubes were open. I felt the doctors there were very dismissive of us because we were the youngest there by far – I was 26 and Peter was 27. But it wasn't as if I was going in there with unexplained infertility; I actually didn't have periods or ovulate. I was prescribed clomiphene (Clomid), and took it for three months, but there was still no sign of either ovulation or a period.

Then Peter was offered a great job in the Netherlands. We decided to move and were pleased to find out his new job included health insurance. The Dutch doctors started by repeating the same fertility tests the English ones had done, as well as checking my thyroid medication was right. Like the UK doctors, they prescribed Clomid, and I took four more courses. Still no ovulation. Next, I was prescribed metformin, which doctors were trialling in the Netherlands for controlling PCOS; they thought it might kick-start my periods. Still no response.

I kept myself on a pretty gruelling treatment schedule, with no time off. And the cultural differences sometimes made it even harder. In the Netherlands, they're not as bothered by nakedness as us Brits. When I had an ultrasound scan – which are always internal using a wand and therefore not pleasant, in any case – there's no screen. I had to walk across the room with nothing on from the waist down. And the doctors don't cover you when you're having the scan, either. I almost cried the first time – but I soon learned to wear a longer top.

Every time I went for a scan to see if my ovaries were responding, I had bad news. The doctor would tell me that the little black areas on the screen, which are supposed to turn into follicles containing eggs, were turning into cysts instead. It would make me feel so down and unwomanly.

I'm very curvy with big boobs – I had a proper bra at the age of 11. I'd think to myself: I look like a woman, but I can't do the one thing that women are meant to do – to produce life. What's the point in having boobs if I'll never feed a baby? What's the point in having hips if they'll never carry a baby? An English colleague used to come over for Sunday lunch, and she'd say to me, 'You're so motherly, you're my home away from home.' And I'd think: I know I'm a motherly person, so why isn't it happening for me?

I'm five foot four, and at the time, I was a size 14/16, but also very fit and strong. I tried to lose weight because the doctors told me it would improve my chances and make my body more receptive to the drugs. First I tried calorie counting, which didn't work, then I did a low-GI eating plan, then I tried the South Beach diet. Peter did it with me, and he lost two or three pounds a week, but I didn't lose one, even though I went to the gym every day and, at the weekends, we'd go on 20-mile bike rides.

People used to laugh at work because I would bring in packed lunches of celery and carrot sticks, perhaps a small ham roll. Then I'd go home to, say, a small plate of sweet potato mash. I remember one doctor telling me off, saying, 'I lost a stone and a half just by watching what I ate'. I tried to show him my food diary, explain my tiny portions, but I don't think he believed me.

The next treatment the doctors recommended was an operation called an ovarian wedge resection, where they cut slices out of the ovaries, which is supposed to balance out your hormones and kick-start ovulation. Although it was a major operation, it seemed like our best chance of success, so we decided I'd have it. I hadn't expected it to affect me so much; it took me at least a couple of weeks to recover. The scar was the same size as a Caesarean and I wasn't allowed to drive or walk much for six weeks. Mummy drove me back to the UK to look after me.

Back in the Netherlands, I was put on Clomid again, but there was still no response from my ovaries. We'd really believed the operation was the answer, and I couldn't deal with the fact that I'd put my body under such massive stress for nothing. Screaming at Peter one night, I told him that our marriage was over. There was part of me that was trying to trick him into leaving me, so I could finally give up trying. At the same time, a bigger part of me had to keep going. I couldn't deny Peter the chance of children. Peter stayed his usual, calm, positive self as I shouted at him.

Next, the doctors started us doing IUI, with the same drugs as are used in IVF. Peter would prepare the syringes, taking the vials out of the fridge and drawing out the right amount. But I still didn't ovulate. After every depressing scan and abandoned cycle, I'd call Peter at work with the news, and often be so upset, I wouldn't be able to speak. There would be a pause while he tried to gather himself together for me. And then he'd say, 'Well, it's not happened this month, but we'll try again.'

After each treatment, I would feel something like period pains because the drugs had made my womb lining grow, and then I'd have to take another drug to shed the lining. Each cycle, the doctors increased the dose and finally, on the third one, I had a follicle that looked mature enough to contain an egg. We were so delighted that we could go ahead with the IUI. In the theatre, the nurse told Peter he could press the syringe with his sperm into me, and so be part of the conception. That made us laugh – it seemed so Dutch.

We were due to do the pregnancy test on Christmas Eve, while staying with my parents, and we really thought this was it – this was our time. There was something poetic about the baby being a Christmas present, something lovely to tell everyone. So I did the test, and the result was negative. That was the only time I've seen Peter crumble. He got in the car and didn't come back for two hours. Later, he told me he'd been driving at crazy speeds. He'd ended up at a shopping centre, where he bought me a beautiful necklace – a silver chain with a little off-centre cross with diamonds.

Our next step was IVF because the doctor said he could give me higher doses of drugs than with IUI. So we had three IVF treatments, but never saw another follicle with potential. I was injecting the maximum dose of drugs, but in the end the doctor told me there was no point in continuing, that my ovaries just didn't work.

It was a hideous time: Peter's dad died and we abandoned our third IVF cycle at the same time. I hadn't had a natural period for four years, only the ones caused by medication.

On a visit to the UK, I started seeing a nutritionist for fertility advice. She told me that non-stop fertility treatments had taken their toll on me. I could see she was right: my hair was in bad condition, my nails were brittle, my skin was dull and dry, and I was still battling with my weight. She told me to switch to organic food, reduce my dairy intake and to eat wild fish, not farmed. She also said I was borderline anaemic, so recommended I take iron as well as a high-dose multivitamin and mineral supplement, plus extra vitamin C and an antioxidant supplement called superoxide dismutase (SOD).

Peter and I started to talk about adoption. Peter said, 'Maybe we're not going to have children of our own, but we can give our love to children who don't have parents or who haven't had enough love.' We realised there was no way we'd be able to adopt in the Netherlands, as our Dutch wasn't good enough.

Peter looked for a new job in the UK, and we went straight into the adoption process here. We passed the initial meetings, and it was only then that we realised we were naive to expect to adopt a baby. The agency was pushing for school-aged children, but I wanted to have a child at home and bond with him or her, so we said no. Then we were asked about sibling groups – would we take a three-year-old and an

18-month-old, for example? We thought it over and decided yes, we could definitely cope with having an instant family.

I started looking for a house with four bedrooms, hopefully for our new family. Meanwhile we were living with my parents and Peter was commuting to his new job.

Still grieving for Peter's dad and for the chance of having my own, biological children, I began to have second thoughts about adoption. Walking the dogs one day, I said to Mummy, 'I'm never going to have that feeling of holding my baby in my arms after giving birth.' And she said, 'No, but you'll have something different. When you take your children home for the first time, it will still be special.' We were both crying, and we carried on walking and talking. Getting all my thoughts out in the open felt very healing.

Later that week, I remember saying to Mummy that I didn't feel myself at all, that I had sore boobs and stomach pains. I assumed it was because my womb lining had built up again, and I needed the drugs that would bring on a period. Used to the whole procedure by then – I had to do a pregnancy test before a doctor would prescribe me the drugs – I jumped in the car and drove down the chemist to pick up a test. It was the day we were due to exchange contracts on our new house, so Mummy and Daddy had champagne ready in the fridge, and Peter was due home half an hour later to drink it.

I ran myself a bath and, as my doctor's appointment was the next morning, I thought I'd do the test straight away. I looked at it, and thought: 'Bloody hell. Two lines have come up.' I checked the instructions and yes, I was pregnant. I was walking around the bathroom naked, thinking: I have to tell Peter; I can't tell my parents first. I can remember smiling so much that my cheeks were aching. I didn't even get into the bath.

I heard Peter's car pulling into the drive, threw on a few clothes and ran downstairs. He must have noticed I was looking odd, as he asked me if I was alright. I said, 'Congratulations on the house.' 'Yes,' he said, 'it is a wonderful house.' Then I said, 'Yes, the perfect house for having a baby.' He held me at arm's length, looked at me and said, 'What did you say?' and I said it again, as I pulled the test out of my pocket and handed it to him. We both started crying and hugging. We told my parents, and Mummy burst into tears. So we had champagne and called my sister and she was screaming down the phone with delight.

I must have had one of my random ovulations, and we'd happened to have sex at exactly the right time. We call Alessandra our little miracle child. My periods came back after she was born – I had three in one year, a record for me – and then, all of a sudden, I was pregnant with Dominic. This is amazing, we both thought – a lovely family. Then, when Dominic was less than nine months, I found myself pregnant yet again! And Sebastian, who's now three months, is an absolutely gorgeous baby too.

We're extremely happy. I adore my children and love being a full-time mum. I do sometimes feel a little greedy, having so much. And I want to blow big, fat raspberries at all the doctors who told us it would never happen!

Q: WHY DO YOU THINK YOU GOT PREGNANT NATURALLY IN THE END?

I do think that, in my case, it was helped along because I stuck to my nutritionist's healthy diet. I could feel that eating that way was making me feel more energetic, and I think it helped my body function better too. It's important to do what you can to stay healthy during and after treatment, as it can take a lot out of your body.

My new diet wasn't about losing weight, it was about getting healthy again. And I think coming back to the UK and having a break from the pressure of treatment helped too. I'd ended up so stressed out from treatment and from the constant hope each time that it might work.

Q: HOW SHOULD YOU CHOOSE THE COMPLEMENTARY THERAPY THAT'S RIGHT FOR YOU?

The nutritionist I saw was very well qualified and her recommendations were based on science, which was important for me. And she was happy to work with my doctors.

I also think that therapies that relax you are a good idea as, at this time, you need all the help you can get, both emotionally and physically. On the other hand, I do know people who've spent a fortune on various therapies with no success. What you should beware of, in my opinion, are therapists who make big claims about getting you pregnant.

Q: HOW CAN YOU STAY EMOTIONALLY HEALTHY WHEN TREATMENT ISN'T WORKING?

Stay positive, as it may happen for you as it did for us. Miracles do happen. My advice – and I wish I'd followed it – is not to make having treatment the be-all and end-all. Make sure you have a life, and that you give yourself time to recover between treatments, so your body and brain can relax. Of course, often couples are under time pressure, so that's not possible.

I think I paid for having continuous treatment by getting unwell. I carried on doing treatments for far too long. Each doctor would say they couldn't do any more for me, but then would refer me on for a different treatment. I shouldn't have kept on until I was so stressed out that I was screaming at my husband to leave me.

• • • • • • • • •

When it comes to natural therapies, it's really important to keep a sense of perspective (not that I always did). IVF is stressful enough without putting more pressure on yourself.

'Of course diet is important, and most of the women I see have a fantastic diet, but there's often a lot of tension around food too, and that's not helpful,' says Emma Cannon. You can't eat a perfect diet, but you can eat a mostly healthy one and not beat yourself up about occasional (or even daily) junk. You can't do every therapy, but you can find one that helps you to relax and a therapist who gets you through the stress of treatment, giving you a sense of control at a time when it may feel as if your body is the property of the medical profession.

Make sure any therapists you go to are accredited by their professional body. One who specialises in fertility is often better, as you don't want to be the one telling *them* how IVF works. According to the 2010 *Red* Annual National Fertility Report, people spend an average of over £1100 on therapies; nearly three quarters of them thought it was money well spent, although a third were worried that some natural fertility treatments are not scientifically proven.

The best therapists work alongside medical doctors, and don't advise you not to have medical treatment. One of the most popular treatments is acupuncture (find an acupuncturist at acupuncture.org.uk or acupuncture-fertility.org), which is also the one with the most studies behind it. Emma Cannon (emmacannon.co.uk), an acupuncturist who specialises in fertility, has written a fertility book from a Chinese medical perspective – *The Baby-Making Bible* (Rodale) – that's based on nurturing yourself. Women I've spoken to also rate hypnosis (see hypnotheraptists.org.uk and Zita West's home hypnotherapy DVDs at zitawest.com), reflexology (aor.org.uk) and herbal medicine (see nimh.org.uk). What's most important is to find a therapy that you like and believe in.

When it comes to eating and supplements, the nutritional scientist Marilyn Glenville keeps her advice up to date on her website marilynglenville.com; also see her book, *Getting Pregnant Faster* (Kyle Cathie). Zita West's own brand of supplements are tailor-made for different stages of conception (see zitawest.com).

Surviving IVF

• • • • • • • • • • • • •

'I want the boys to be proud of how they were made. It's important not to be ashamed of IVF.'

'I wish I could have stepped outside of myself for five minutes and seen how out of control I was getting, and what it was doing to us.'

'It's so painful when you're going through infertility. But now Sumaya is eight months old, I feel I've got to a place where I can look back on what happened. I'm delighted to have a daughter. But I still feel sad and cheated that I didn't experience falling pregnant naturally.'

'Although IVF is tough on both of you, mentally and emotionally, try to do things together in your relationship that you always liked, so there's some kind of normality.'

'It isn't easy. It's a journey with lots of twists and turns, but I'd do it again, without doubt.'

My twin IVF pregnancy

• • • • • • • • • • • •

Despite the fact that all UK IVF clinics now follow the official guidelines for reducing the number of multiple pregnancies, your chance of an IVF pregnancy being twins or more is just over one in five, according to figures from 2009 (compared to a chance of one in 80 if you conceive naturally).

There are a few reasons why the odds are still relatively high, despite the single embryo transfer policy (see Chapter 10): you can still have two embryos put back on your second cycle, if your first was unsuccessful; and, if you're 40 or over, you can have three put back.

The majority of IVF twins are 'fraternal', that is they come from two separate embryos, so are only genetically as close as any brother or sister. But there is also a slightly higher incidence of identical twins from fertility treatment: 'After transfer of blastocysts [embryos grown in the lab for five days], and also after ICSI, there is evidence of a slightly higher rate of division,' says Jane Denton, Director of the

Multiple Births Foundation – in other words, the embryo splits and the twins have the same genetic make-up. 'Now more blastocyst transfers are being done, we can see the result in the pregnancies.' And, she warns, because an embryo can split, a single one can turn into twins, but two embryos could become triplets with one identical pair, or even quads.

One crucial detail you should find out, says Denton, is whether twin babies share a placenta (which only happens with identical twins). 'If they do, monitoring of the pregnancy will be more intensive because there's a risk of twin-to-twin syndrome – an imbalance in the blood flow between the babies, so one has more than the other.'

With multiples, the statistics can seem scary – the risk of stillbirth, for example, is more than double with twins – and although the majority of twin pregnancies do go well, with no lasting health problems for mother or baby, the challenges of parenting twins are often underestimated, according to Denton.

As someone who's doubly pregnant, you can reduce the risks that come with getting bigger than the average pregnancy with some advice from a physiotherapist. 'Being taught how to sit, stand, sleep and walk, so that you avoid any back strain or other long-term effects should be a routine part of maternity care,' says Denton. Nicola, 43, mother to three-year-old twins Florence and Mabel, had to have an operation for her back pain. 'I had a crushed disc that was pressing on the nerves that went down my leg. It was so painful, I could hardly walk. The doctor said I'd put my back under a lot more wear and tear than it would normally have had, being pregnant with two babies, then picking them up and carrying them around for the first two years too.'

Finally, twins are often delivered early – 37 weeks is considered full term, and over half come before then – so your planning needs to be done early too. 'We advise mothers to start antenatal classes at around 24 weeks,' says Denton.

● ● ● ● ● ● ● ●

Sarah, a full-time mum from the West Midlands, was 28 when she had IVF and got pregnant with twin boys.

Our boys were born at 31 weeks, by emergency C-section. I'd been given a sedative during the operation because they'd had to get the babies out quickly before my epidural had had a chance to work; so by the time I woke up, it was four hours after the birth.

The nurses wanted to take me up to the ward straight away, but I wanted to see the babies. My husband Carl hadn't been allowed to touch the babies when they were born, but he'd glimpsed them across the operating theatre before they were taken up to the special-care baby unit (SCBU), and all he'd been told was that he had two sons.

Carl asked the nurse for a wheelchair, and wheeled me down to see the boys in the SCBU. It was quite dark and very warm – 30 degrees. It wasn't bare and clinical as I'd expected – there were bright curtains with an animal print and lots of toys. The boys were lying in incubators, next to each other. The first thing I noticed was how tiny they were – just 30cm long. One weighed 3lb 12oz and the other weighed 3lb 10oz. Their thighs were the length of my thumb, and the back of their hands was the same size as my thumbnail. Their nappies were the smallest size you can buy, but they still came up to their chins.

It was quite scary and shocking, as they were in the intensive-care section of the SCBU. They were in incubators with heart and oxygen monitors, drips in their hands and nasal feeding tubes; all kinds of wires and cables were coming out of them, with the machines making bleeping sounds. Luckily, they were breathing well, so they didn't need to be on ventilators.

We couldn't pick up the babies or cuddle them, so we just looked at them. I was still woozy from the drugs, so didn't get upset, but I remember saying, straight away, 'That one's Damien, and that one's Daegan'.

It was only later that day, when I was on the ward, that I realised the full implications of them being so tiny. I knew I wouldn't be taking them home straight away. I asked a nurse, and she said, 'You'll be lucky to get them home before your due date.' That horrified me: I hadn't realised that it could be so long. In the end, I was in hospital for a week, and they were in for four. But as long as the boys were doing well, I was happy. It had taken us three cycles of IVF with ICSI to conceive them, after all.

Our problem had seemed simple at first: Carl had had a vasectomy – he'd been married before and was already a dad to two girls. Because the vasectomy was relatively recent, only a year before we met, his doctor thought there was a very good chance that the vasectomy reversal would be successful, but it wasn't. Apparently, a vasectomy can affect the quality of the sperm.

Once we saw the sperm analysis in black and white, it was pretty obvious that ICSI was the only way we'd have children together. I was happy to be a stepmum, but I didn't want only to be a stepmum. The girls, who were then eight and 10, came to stay every other weekend, which meant we did lovely family things, but it also reminded me I didn't have my own children. I come from a very close family and the thought of growing old without children and grandchildren was awful.

To start with, I found having IVF exciting, the fact we were doing something positive to get pregnant. With the first cycle, I had nine eggs collected, and the embryologists used ICSI to make seven embryos. There were only two good ones left when I had them put back in, but I got pregnant. We were so excited, talking about whether the baby was going to be a boy or a girl, planning our future. Then, at five and a half weeks, I miscarried.

Carl and I hadn't told anyone we were having IVF; we were going to keep it secret until after the 12-week scan. But after I started bleeding, I spent the whole afternoon and evening crying, and we ended up telling our families not only that we'd had IVF but that I'd had a miscarriage too. My mum was really upset that I'd gone through so much without confiding in her. I explained that because we'd thought it would work, we'd assumed we could do it on our own.

We waited the recommended three months before we tried again but, looking back, it wasn't long enough. I think I was depressed. Everyone around us seemed to be getting pregnant: I counted 22 babies conceived by friends and family while we were trying. For three months, I just went to work and came home, and thought: that's another day closer to getting pregnant.

I was negative all through the next cycle. We did get 11 eggs, and 10 fertilised, but again, we only had two left when it came to transfer. I didn't feel pregnant at all during the two-week wait – just blank and vacant – and I was right. We decided not to have another cycle for six months and to have a really cracking Christmas and New Year, with a few too many drinks.

I felt mentally and emotionally ready for our third cycle. And it worked! Almost from the day of the pregnancy test, I felt shocking – physically sick from the moment I opened my eyes to bedtime. I used to come home from work and fall asleep on the sofa. I'd put on weight having IVF – around a stone – but I lost it all in the first couple of weeks, going back to eight stone, as I could hardly eat.

I didn't know of anybody having twins, and it just hadn't occurred to me that we'd have them, even after having had two embryos put back. At the six-week scan, when the sonographer pointed out the second heartbeat, I was emotional, crying with joy. Carl was so shocked he couldn't speak for the next two hours.

I was wearing maternity clothes before my eight-week scan. I'm only five foot one, and I got big very quickly. I loved every minute of being pregnant. But by 31 weeks, I was enormous, and my tummy skin was shiny and could hardly stretch any more. I think I went into labour purely because there wasn't any more room!

When my waters broke, I went to hospital and they took me into theatre to deliver, just in case there were complications. Once it started to really hurt, they gave me an epidural, but within 10 minutes Daegan's heart rate had dropped, and that's when they operated. I remember excruciating pain, as the epidural hadn't kicked in, then nothing, because the anaesthetist knocked me out.

The day after the boys were born, I was allowed to hold them, which was amazing and scary at the same time. They seemed so fragile and light and there were so many wires connected to them. The nurses taught me what all the monitors did and, once I'd held the boys a few times, I was confident that I could get them out of the incubators myself. Bleeping meant everything was fine, but when the heart rate monitor bleeped frantically it meant the baby's heart rate had dropped. Then, you had to give the baby a gentle shake or rub him on the back.

Eventually, even though there was so much noise from the machines, the SCBU seemed really quiet. I spent all the time I could with the boys. After I was discharged, Carl and I got into a routine, coming in every day, sitting and talking to the boys, stroking their hands. I'd get to the hospital before nine in the morning, then leave at eleven-thirty, go home and express some milk, go back in at one, then go home at six. I was exhausted as, to keep my milk flowing, I was expressing at 2 a.m. too.

The twins weren't allowed to come home before they were feeding properly, so I spent two weeks trying to get them to latch on and breastfeed. Eventually, I managed a full day of feeding them, then a full night. That was the first time I learned to pick them up and feed them together. It was a challenge, but it was an adrenaline kick to have both my babies to myself for the first time. And, the next day, they were allowed home, which was amazing.

When they left the hospital, Daegan was just over 4lb and Damien was 4lb 6oz. They didn't cry or murmur – they were still like newborns. It was a milestone when they reached 5lb, then 6lb, but I soon forgot how small they'd been. Now they're three, they're running around like crazy and they're huge. They look completely different from each other: Damien is stockier and taller with mousy hair; Daegan is blond and smaller, but extra loud. They've got a very strong bond – they do fight, but they look after each other too.

Q: WHAT'S YOUR VIEW ON THE SINGLE EMBRYO TRANSFER POLICY?

I don't regret having two embryos put back. I think if you pay all that money for IVF, you've worked hard to save it and you've gone on that emotional rollercoaster, I think you should have the choice.

I know there's a concern about multiple pregnancies and the health of the babies, but the year I got pregnant, I met seven other sets of twins conceived through IVF, and though all except one set came early, they're all healthy and doing well. If I'd heard any negative stories about people having twins, then perhaps I'd feel differently, but I haven't.

Now I've had my boys, I wouldn't change it. Because I had two children at once, I don't want any more and I feel our family is complete, whereas if I'd had one baby, I would probably want to have IVF again, to try for a second child. And I'm not sure if my husband would agree to that.

Q: WILL YOU TELL THE TWINS HOW THEY WERE CONCEIVED?

I want the boys to be proud of how they were made. It's important not to be ashamed of IVF. If anyone asks me if twins run in the family, I'm proud to tell them that the boys were created in a lab. In fact, we nicknamed them Frank and Stein when they were in the womb! IVF doesn't mean you're any different; just that you need some help with conceiving.

Q: WHAT'S YOUR ADVICE TO ANYONE WHO FINDS OUT SHE'S PREGNANT WITH TWINS?

Don't panic! Even though you might read so many statistics about twin pregnancies going wrong, don't spend your whole pregnancy worrying. Try to enjoy being pregnant, if you can. I enjoyed it to the max.

Reading accounts of other people's pregnancies and births helped to put my mind at rest over whether I'd cope. I read Dr Carol Cooper's book [see below for details]. I also looked at the TAMBA website and made contact with other women who had got pregnant with twins at the same time, via my IVF clinic forum.

I didn't plan the birth, as the boys were so early. But I think you're only going to be disappointed if you have a rigid birth plan with twins. From the 12-week scan onwards, I started organising the essentials: car seats, pushchair, Moses baskets, clothes, sheets. I'd say buy just what you need, no more. Twins are expensive.

· · · · · · · · ·

The Multiple Births Foundation (MBF, at multiplebirths.org. uk and 020 3313 3519) is a charity that supports families with twins and triplets, as well as training professionals to provide support. Their website is the place to go for medical information; there are leaflets on preparing for twins, on twins who share a placenta, on breastfeeding and sleep, all written by experts in the field. There is also information on a subject that's often taboo: reducing the number of foetuses. 'We are a point of contact for any queries you may have about your twin or more pregnancy, any questions to which you aren't finding the answers,' says Jane Denton.

Both the MBF and its sister organisation Twins and Multiple Births Association (TAMBA) run courses for expectant parents. TAMBA is the twin and multiples charity organised by parents. They have a phone help and support line (Twinline – 0800 138 0509; it's open from 10 a.m. to 1 p.m. and 7 p.m. to 10 p.m.), although you should consult your doctor about any medical questions.

TAMBA also runs a network of twins clubs (details at tamba.org.uk). There are non-affiliated twins clubs, too (see twinsclubs.org.uk). Christina Tyson, a mum of twins who runs the North West London twins club, says that other parents are a very good source of practical advice on multiple parenting, from breastfeeding and sleep routines to helping you find out about equipment. 'People are really good at freaking you out,' she says. 'In fact, you wouldn't be normal if you weren't freaked out. My advice is: never take advice from women who've only got one baby!' She recommends reading *Baby Secrets: How to Know Your Baby's Needs* by Jo Tantum and Barbara Want (Michael Joseph), for advice on routines, and Emma Mahony's *Double Trouble: Twins and How To Survive Them* (Thorsons). 'It's quite fun and easy to read,' she says. For good all-round advice, read twin expert and GP Dr Carol Cooper's *Twins & Multiple Births: The Essential Parenting Guide From Pregnancy to Adulthood* (Vermilion).

IVF could have ended my relationship

· · · · · · · · · · · ·

Often, IVF can put a strain on relationships, leading to arguments and even break-ups. Zita West runs a natural and assisted-conception fertility clinic in London that provides relationship counselling. 'When a couple goes through IVF the first time, it's a novel experience, and often their relationship is loving and supportive. But by the time they get to their third or even fifth or sixth go, it's not unusual for the relationship to have started to deteriorate. They may have stopped having sex now they're doing IVF. Typically, the man worries about the money, while the woman worries about taking time off work. And the cracks can really start to show when one partner – usually the woman – wants to keep going with treatment, and the other doesn't.'

Personally, I've found that fertility issues have sometimes brought my husband and I closer together, while other times they've led to our most ferocious arguments. He says he wasn't properly consulted before I booked in for our second cycle. I think the problem was, as Zita says, that I was focused only on treatment. At that point, I was having so many conversations with experts, therapists and friends, that I didn't talk to him properly.

Fertility coach, Anya Sizer often sees a similar pattern, with one partner racing ahead of the other when it comes to planning the next IVF cycle, or switching to a different treatment. 'You have to accept that's normal, and go with the partner who's at the slowest pace. And don't expect to get all your support from each other. Fertility treatment puts an enormous strain on all couples, and outside support, whether it's friends, family or counselling, is very helpful.'

Also, with those whose quest for a baby has lasted years, Anya says that the couple can turn into people going through treatment, rather than a couple. 'It can become very easy that the only thing you talk about is fertility. Instead, try to be a couple together again, and to have a life outside fertility.'

●　●　●　●　●　●　●　●　●

For Sam, 39, a magazine editor from London, having a baby became an obsession that almost ended her relationship with her husband David.

For me, IVF was like an addiction to lottery tickets; as soon as I knew I'd lost, I wanted another one. I became obsessed by it, I just wanted more and I didn't care how I was going to get it.

After my second IVF treatment failed, I started looking online at egg donation, thinking: well, let's try that now. I got into a terrible habit of going in chat rooms all the time and seeing what treatment other women were having. Reading about one couple who'd had IVF 15 times, I thought of it not as an awful trial, but as a badge of honour.

I started looking into adoption too. My mind was running at a million miles an hour, not considering what David was thinking. I thought, as we can afford it, I'll do anything to have a baby.

But we didn't have unlimited money, and I never thought about the pressure I was putting on David. I only found out later that the more I talked to him about fertility treatment, the more he felt he couldn't make me happy because he couldn't give me the baby I wanted so much.

It was on my birthday, a few months after the second IVF failed, that David said he couldn't handle being with me any more. I'd managed to get front-row tickets to see Neil Young, who's a real hero of ours. On the underground going home, David said, out of the blue, 'I really need to get away from you for a few weeks'. I hadn't seen it coming, I was so caught up in all the madness of IVF. I knew we weren't getting on, but he was supposed to be the strong one, not the one being affected, like me.

I'd never considered that having children would be hard when we got married, three years before. I was so naive; I thought we'd just decide to have children, then they'd come along.

A few months after the wedding, we went on a romantic long weekend to Morocco. After a night in Marrakech, we drove for a couple of hours to an incredible retreat – a riad in the middle of the desert; the gardens were cool, lush and green, an oasis, with hammocks and palm trees. It was a really hot day and, on arriving, I felt a bit dizzy and strange, so I sat down to rest under the trees. I don't know why I felt my leg, but suddenly my fingers picked out a lump at the top, in my groin. At first, I assumed it was an insect bite but it was big, the size of a golf ball.

David thought I should get it checked out by a doctor, so we drove back to Marrakech. The doctor gave me an ultrasound scan. Then, via my limited French and his little English, he told me I had a huge 'tumour', that it was 'very serious' and that I needed to fly home immediately. I could only assume that by 'tumour', he meant it was cancer. David and I were beside ourselves, crying on the way back to the hotel. We took the first available flight home.

Back in the UK, my GP referred me to a gynaecologist. He was 95 per cent certain that the lump wasn't cancer, but a really, really large fibroid – bigger than a grapefruit – on the outside of my womb, with one of its ends growing rapidly into my groin. Fibroids are very common, but it's pretty unusual for one to be so big. I couldn't believe I had something so huge inside me. I had noticed my stomach had got rounder, but just thought I needed to do a few sit-ups.

The doctor said I needed to have the fibroid removed, but assured me it wouldn't affect my fertility. It was frightening having the operation, especially as, with my case being so unusual, there were lots of medical students watching. The surgeon operated through an incision the same as a C-section. Fully revealed, the fibroid turned out to be 10cm long. They had to pull it out with forceps, like a baby, because it had started to rot and was stuck fast. It was a long operation; I lost four pints of blood.

When I woke up, the doctor told me that the fibroid had grown around my Fallopian tubes. He said one was broken, and the other was blocked, so it could affect my chances of getting pregnant, although the blocked one might open itself again.

It took me around four months to get back to normal from the operation. I was 35 by this time, and realised that if we wanted babies, we should start trying straight away. I bought ovulation kits and – I can see with hindsight – started to get slightly obsessive, putting pressure on David to have sex when I was ovulating. Every month, I assumed we'd get a positive pregnancy result, and then we didn't. Five months on, I went back to the doctor who had done the operation. He advised us to go straight for IVF.

I thought: brilliant, a solution; now we can just get on with having a baby. I persuaded David we shouldn't wait to get to the top of the long NHS waiting list, but should just go to a good clinic and get it over with. We chose the ARGC.

At first, IVF felt like a little project that we had to get through. I remember when I had to do my first injection, I was even excited. You have to give almost your whole life over to the ARGC, because there are blood tests every morning, as well as regular scans. I was working, which made it hard when they called me, sometimes in the middle of the day, to tell me to come to the clinic straight away. And usually, I'd have to wait, as there were so many other women there too. Nobody at work knew I was having IVF, so I had to make up all kinds of excuses to get to clinic appointments.

Even though I was being monitored constantly by the clinic, emotionally I felt lost and confused. But the doctors said my case – damaged tubes – was straightforward, which meant that I had a very good chance.

On the first cycle, I produced 15 eggs and 12 of them fertilised with David's sperm, which was great. But by day five after egg collection, we only had two embryos which were of good enough quality. That was disappointing, as I'd hoped to freeze some for the next baby. I started to feel under pressure. We'd extended our mortgage by £15,000 to pay for treatment. We'd assumed that would be enough to pay for three rounds, but at the ARGC the first round cost £8000.

About eight days after embryo transfer, I started to bleed. I was so upset. I called the clinic and they told me to wait and then do my pregnancy blood test on the correct day. On the day of the test, I waited for my results in the clinic, still bleeding heavily. It felt like every woman in there was pregnant except me. Later that day, I got a call saying my beta hCG level was 58, which is, officially, pregnant, but they prefer it to be at least 100.

That's when the madness really started. I had to go to the clinic every other day to make sure my levels were doubling – and they were, at first. I was still bleeding and I didn't feel pregnant physically, but I did in my mind. The clinic told me that low beta hCG levels can sometimes be a proper pregnancy. Suddenly, 10 days later, they told me my levels were looking strange and to come in for a scan the next day. They had a look at the embryo, and said it looked small, but to come back in a week.

Then, when there was still no heartbeat, the doctor said that he was very sorry, but it definitely wasn't going to progress. He asked me what I wanted to do, but I didn't have a clue what he meant. He explained I could go home and let things take their course – pass the pregnancy naturally – or go to the hospital and have it removed. I decided to go home as, frankly, I'd had enough of medicine and doctors.

That was a very strange time – waiting for the miscarriage. The pain and bleeding started three days later at work. Then, that night, when I went to the loo at my sister's, I saw a little grey sac, which was really shocking. I had to pull it out as it had got stuck. I wish someone had told me I'd actually see what could have been our baby – that it was going to be horrible and upsetting. It was too much to cope with for both of us; we were so upset. Later on, I was pleased I hadn't been to hospital, so I'd been able to keep the sac. We buried it under a tree in our garden.

I'd been so busy trying to get and stay pregnant, then, all of sudden, there was nothing. I didn't know how to cope. The grief didn't go away, but after a couple of weeks I started to think of the miscarriage as just bad luck. The doctors say it happens a lot to people on their first time. So I thought: fine, we'll give it another go.

By this time, I was 36 and panicking about running out of time, so two months later, we were back in the clinic. I can see now that we didn't give ourselves enough of a break. Suddenly, our lives were all about making a baby. Everything that was fun, like going out after work and seeing friends, became impossible because we'd hardly told anyone we were doing IVF. I wasn't drinking and I didn't want to be out late, so I became increasingly isolated.

I went to see an acupuncturist who insisted she should treat David too. She gave us Chinese herbs to boil up and make into tea to drink every day. He hated it. His sperm was fine, so he couldn't understand why I was making him do this. We were also under double pressure: emotionally and financially. This time, it felt as if IVF had to work.

Yet again, we got another positive pregnancy test, and it all started again – the blood tests and scans. Before transfer, the ARGC had advised us to have immune testing – reproductive immunology is controversial, but something that they specialise in. My blood tests came back positive, so I was advised to have a treatment called IVIg (intravenous immunoglobulin). It's a blood product, administered via a drip into a vein, that's supposed to prevent your immune system from rejecting the embryo. I had one IVIg during treatment, then three more after I got pregnant. It's not cheap and the cycle added up to nearly £10,000.

Then, at the seven-week scan, we saw a heartbeat, which was a huge relief. The doctor said the embryo was quite small, but I thought it would all be fine and became quite relaxed at my weekly scans. But when I went for one at 10 weeks, the doctor said, 'I'm really sorry, the heartbeat has gone'. As I was walking down the stairs, one of the nurses asked me if everything was all right, and I had to say, 'No, actually it's not', in front of the other patients. I was trying so hard to keep it together. I remember walking out on to the street and thinking: what do I do now? I called David and went down a little side street and cried and cried.

I couldn't cope with waiting for the miscarriage again, so I went straight into hospital to have the pregnancy taken out with an ERPC under general anaesthetic. I was totally hysterical and didn't know what to do with myself. I'd kept in all my emotions after the first miscarriage, then everything came out all at once while I was being wheeled down to theatre. I couldn't even breathe, I was crying so much. I couldn't deal with the end of another potential baby. The same doctor who had operated on my fibroid did the ERPC. He and the nurses were so kind and understanding. I asked them to put me out straight away.

David and I were in different places for quite a while after that. At first, he was very caring. I wanted to go straight back to the clinic for another cycle, but he kept saying we should think about the money. And I'd reply, 'I don't care how much it costs. If it costs a million pounds, I'll find it.' I was in total meltdown for weeks. I lost all interest in anything I enjoyed, cried all the time I was at home, only just managing to keep it together at work. David did the typical male thing of not talking to anyone about the miscarriage, pretending it hadn't happened.

It wasn't so much that we had lost a baby – although that did hurt. It was more that I was wondering what my life was going to be like. Would I have to have IVF every few months? Go through this again and again? My life seemed to be all about doctors' appointments and tests. I'd come home from work, and all my conversation would be about fertility. I forgot how to talk about anything else.

Another reason why our relationship started to unravel was because we hadn't told many people. Our families knew something was up, but not that we were having IVF. Good friends of mine tried to be supportive, but they didn't really understand what you go through with IVF. So it was easier to keep it to myself. No one at work knew. It was embarrassing to talk about IVF because it felt as if we'd failed. I didn't want people to feel sorry for us. And if you tell people you're trying, when it fails you have to explain that you're not pregnant.

So we only had each other. David didn't want to talk about it and I wanted to talk about it all the time. The baby issue became the elephant in the room. We started taking things out on each other. I actually started to hate him.

We were like that for a whole year. We can talk about it quite openly now, but we very nearly broke up. Instead of becoming closer, we became distant and dealt with the situation in different ways. We'd try to go out together for dinner and, every time, I'd get really upset and he'd get angry. Where we live is nappy valley, so I'd see pregnant women all the time, reminding me of the potential children I had lost, and the ones I might never have. I went from being a fun person, full of life, to being weak and vulnerable. And I couldn't see how to change back again.

When David did talk about IVF, he said we had to get on with life, not just think about babies. But I thought: how can I have a life without a baby in it? That Christmas, we argued all the time. I was on the internet constantly, looking at different clinics, adoption in the UK, adoption abroad – anything for a baby.

It was a few months after this that David told me he wanted time apart. In the end, it was me who moved out. I went to stay with a friend for six weeks. I did move back in after that, but we weren't back together properly. It was a dreadful summer because I was so scared of losing David that I tried to become the perfect partner: I never argued or brought up babies or IVF in conversation any more. But I was trying to be somebody I wasn't, and that couldn't last. Finally, I realised I had to be honest and not tread on eggshells around him any more. So I told him that if he didn't want to be with me, I didn't care any more, but that he had to make the decision.

David was so shocked, he had to go out for a walk to think. Afterwards, he said he realised that he did want to be with me. But even after that, we didn't go back to being close. I kept thinking, how could he want to split up, then assume that everything was back to normal? We still weren't discussing IVF or babies. But one night, at dinner, David apologised to my parents for what he'd put me through. He didn't say sorry directly to me, though I knew he was trying to make up for what had happened because he was being so considerate and kind.

It was only in September, when our names finally came up for IVF on the NHS, that we had to start talking about it again. We couldn't agree: I wanted to go ahead, and David wasn't sure. Even on the day I was given the drugs to start, I came home and asked him if we were going to do it. I knew I couldn't do it without his support, however much I wanted a baby.

David said, 'Ok, let's try and see what happens.' So we did, and it didn't work. I thought that would be the end of us. But it was David who encouraged me to try again. He was suddenly supportive. I think he'd finally realised that if we didn't have IVF, we might never have a family.

We changed to a different clinic, where the treatment was much more relaxed as we saw the same nurse at every appointment. When the time came for the pregnancy test, I didn't want to do it. Even when I got a positive result, I was convinced it would end in miscarriage. Then I went for the blood test and had ridiculously high levels of beta hCG – about 600 – and realised I really was properly pregnant this time.

The whole nine months, I never took my pregnancy for granted. I bled every three to four weeks, and ended up in A&E getting checked out every time. Having Lenny is incredible and everything I expected it to be and more. He's nearly a year old now. He's been such a good baby and sleeps through the night, but if there's any chance of anything going wrong, I'm overcautious. I know all new mums are like that, but I think I'm much worse because it was so hard to conceive him.

Even after Lenny was born, my feeling of inadequacy due to not being able to get pregnant stayed with me. I felt like an infiltrator at the new-mum groups – as if I hadn't earned my place the same way as everyone else. Then, when Lenny was six months, we were completely shocked to find out that I was pregnant. I even said to my GP, 'Could there be any other reason than a baby for a positive pregnancy test?'

Now, I'm seven months pregnant, and the new baby finally feels real. I'm so happy to be in this incredible position. But, funnily enough, it's only now that I can look back and see that our life could have been great without children too.

Q: WHY DO YOU THINK IVF PUTS SUCH A STRAIN ON RELATIONSHIPS?

Firstly, there's so much riding on it. It's all about your hopes, ambitions and dreams for your family, and none of it is under your control. It's down to chance, a throw of the dice.

Secondly, it's much more pressured for the woman, as it's her body, and she's more likely to get into the whole process and need to know more about it. David was much more removed from it, and would always say, like a lot of men, that everything was going to be fine. He wanted us to enjoy ourselves and not think about IVF, and IVF was all I wanted to think about.

Q: HOW COULD YOU HAVE SUPPORTED YOUR RELATIONSHIP?

I can't see how – unless it works first time – any couple going through IVF could avoid going on some sort of journey together. It does make you contemplate the big questions in life. Other couples don't often get tested like that, especially relatively early in a relationship. One minute we were on honeymoon, the next we were debating if we were ever going to have children, and what old age would be like without them. For people to come through IVF and still be together says a lot for their relationship.

At the time, we thought it was a good idea not to tell many people, to cut the stress of being asked about it. But that turned out to be the worst idea ever, as we only had each other to talk to. So I think getting support from other people is essential; ideally, someone who understands or who has been through IVF. So many people are doing it now, but people still talk about it in hushed tones. The more you are open about it, the more others who are going through it will feel as if it's normal.

Q: DO YOU HAVE ANY REGRETS ABOUT WHAT HAPPENED BETWEEN YOU AND YOUR PARTNER?

I should have been kinder to him. I got caught up in the world of infertility. I couldn't bear to be the person who was going to end up without children, so I decided to do whatever it took. I didn't really have a life for four years. And so I left David behind. If I could have got a loan for £100,000, I would have taken it and not thought twice about it. I didn't care about the financial position I was putting both of us in. I wish I could have stepped outside of myself for five minutes and seen how out of control I was getting, and what it was doing to us.

• • • • • • • • •

According to the 2010 *Red* Annual National Fertility Report, 25 per cent of women who'd had fertility problems said their sex life suffered and 6 per cent split up because of difficulty trying to conceive. The women also said that for a third of couples, it was the man who coped less well with fertility treatment.

Once you realise that you can't expect your partner to be thinking exactly the same way as you are about treatment at exactly the same time, it can become easier, according to Anya Sizer. She has a chapter on keeping your relationship strong in her book, *Fertile Thinking* (Infinite Ideas). Her website is thefertilitycoach.co.uk.

Zita West's clinic also provide couples' counselling (zitawest.com) in London. Nationwide, the specialist fertility counsellors at bica.net are used to the issues that come up in infertility, but there are also other organisations of counsellors and therapists: bacp.co.uk, psychotherapy.org.uk and bps.org.uk. Relate are the most famous couples' therapy organisation (relate.org.uk), plus they're a charity, so the fees can be less than with a private therapist. The most important thing is to find someone you want to talk to and who suits you.

If you prefer to read a book, I found the approach of the US family therapist, M. Gary Neuman, eye-opening. His books aren't aimed at couples going through infertility, but, *In Good Times & Bad* (John Wiley & Sons) has a section on strengthening your relationship (if you can bear to ignore the section on how to decrease the effects of stress on children) and *Connect to Love* (also Wiley) is a two-week programme on relationship strengthening. The biggest lesson I learned is that even if one person – i.e. you – changes his or her attitude, the relationship can become less stressful.

Therapy got me through IVF

• • • • • • • • • • • •

I f you had a broken-down boiler or a dodgy clutch, you'd call in the professionals. So why not do that when it comes to your emotional health? Most IVF clinics either have their own counsellor or can recommend one. Even so, according to Mollie Graneek, a specialist fertility counsellor, some people are still reluctant to seek help: 'People often have negative perceptions of counselling, as if it's an admission of failure. That can compound their feelings about their "failure" to conceive. Most people have been brought up to believe that asking for help is a sign of weakness.'

What surprised me about counselling is how unlike the cliché of therapy it is. There's no delving into your past, digging up the reasons for your emotions. Instead, the counsellor was more like a sounding board, helping me to describe what I was feeling after my miscarriage, and telling me that my emotions were normal, considering what I'd been through.

'Counselling may help you through a time of crisis', says Graneek, 'and help you get insight into your feelings. A counsellor will give you support and empathy, and accept your painful feelings in a non-judgmental way.'

Not being able to get pregnant – or the failure of an IVF cycle – can bring up a whole spectrum of negative feelings, from anger and sadness to grief and guilt. 'When a woman cannot conceive, she often convinces herself that something is wrong with her, that she must have done something bad to "deserve" this. She may feel ashamed, or that she's fundamentally different from other women,' says Graneek.

She adds that the diagnosis of infertility can, very often, begin to define who you are. Friends and family who don't know what to say can become guarded, or you could feel they're being patronising. 'And diagnosis also brings with it a sense of loss and grief that's hard to explain. After all, how can you grieve what you've never had? Then there is guilt – the feeling of letting someone down, whether it's your partner or parents. And, of course anger, asking, "Why me?"

'When people experience these strong, difficult feelings, they very often disown them, saying things like, "I'm not usually like this" or "I don't want to feel like this" or "I feel out of control." Counselling can help you to reconcile your feelings, and come to terms with this new and difficult side of yourself.'

● ● ● ● ● ● ● ●

Oona, 43, a parenting psychologist from London, knew she needed professional support in order to get through IVF.

I always tried so hard to keep it together at work but, that day, I only just managed to stop myself from crying. I was teaching a group parenting class for mothers who were having problems loving and taking care of their children. I had tried to help one woman to understand her negative feelings, but she'd thrown it back at me. 'You don't have any kids, so how the hell would you know?' she'd said. She'd kept on making comments like that for the rest of the session. When I left the class, I sobbed all the way home on the bus, collapsing when I got inside.

I'm trained as a counsellor and psychologist, and I specialise in parenting – ante- and postnatal. So at work, I deal with anything from parenting problems, to having lost a baby, to coping with twins. Being a mother – or not being one – was always in my face. When I started my job, it was very fulfilling and felt natural to me. I've always had a lot to do with children – growing up in an Irish household you're surrounded by them – and I've always been close to the children of my friends.

It wasn't until I was 37, after Said and I had been married four years, that we started to try seriously for children. I expected to get pregnant quickly, but after nine months, we went to the GP, who sent us for tests. All my results were fine, but we discovered that Said had a low sperm count. So then we knew it wasn't going to be easy to get pregnant.

I'd always thought of myself as an earth mother type. At work, I even taught other mothers *how* to be mothers. I knew I was good at that, but not being able to get pregnant began to make me feel like a fake at work. The reality was, I couldn't be a mother, despite my job. It was a massive blow to my self-esteem.

I couldn't talk about being infertile or own up to it. I come from a big family in Ireland and my husband's family is from Algeria, and he has eleven brothers and sisters. So there were massive expectations from both of our families. In his culture, it's unheard of to be married for so many years, and not to have a baby. The only thing my mother-in-law could say in English was 'Baby?', and she'd say that every time we stepped off the plane.

On one visit, Said's sister took me aside and asked me why I hadn't got pregnant. I felt so ashamed, as though I wasn't doing the thing I should be doing as a woman. I knew his family would never have begun to understand that it might have been a male problem. Said struggled with that too. As it turned out later on, I had problems as well, but, to this day, he won't entertain the fact that his sperm count contributed at all to our difficulties.

Said and I talked about our options for treatment. He is a Muslim and, at first, he thought that having IVF would be going against God. But I'd converted to Islam when we married, so I was able to discuss the religious arguments with him. There is actually a very positive justification for IVF in Islam: there's an idea that when you have a sickness, you should have a cure; and if infertility is the sickness, IVF is the cure. It's not considered a sin to create embryos outside of the body, as the soul isn't blown into the foetus until you're 120 days pregnant. It's very different from the Roman Catholic beliefs that I grew up with, where the only right way to make a baby is a husband and wife 'lying together'.

A friend who had had IVF recommended the ARGC in London. When we went for our first appointment, the doctor we met was Muslim, and he spoke Arabic to Said. But Said still didn't feel comfortable.

Not being able to conceive became more and more difficult to bear. At the time, everyone around me seemed to be getting pregnant. My younger sister even announced her second pregnancy. I felt totally alone, with no one to talk to.

Around this time, my sister and I took my mum to Paris for her 60th birthday. In a restaurant one evening, we got into a silly argument. Mum was taking my sister's side, and I said, sarcastically, 'Oh yeah, take the side of the pregnant person, she has to be right.' My sister left, upset, and Mum told me that she'd had some spotting the night before, and said that getting and being pregnant isn't easy for anyone. I got really angry; I was even swearing. Then I shouted, 'At least she can *get* pregnant,' and ran out of the restaurant. Outside, I had a massive panic attack, which was extremely frightening. I've never behaved like that before. My emotions were out of control.

I needed someone I could talk to, to clear my head. I had one session with my old therapist, but came away feeling absolutely shattered. I didn't have the stamina to go into depth about every issue. I needed my reserves just to get through the treatment and deal with my stressful job. So it was a deliberate choice to go to see Anya Sizer, who is a fertility coach, not a therapist. I liked the coaching philosophy – that it's about creating attainable goals, looking at how you've coped before and using that to build strategies. I wanted to see someone who was experienced in fertility treatment too. And who wasn't going to need a commitment to a weekly face-to-face meeting. I knew how many clinic appointments I'd have to fit in while having IVF, and I didn't want to add in yet another one. With Anya, I could do our session on the phone, or even get her feedback by email or text.

Because of my job, I'm often the one to whom friends turn for advice. So when I saw Anya, it was a relief to take off my expert's hat, and just be Oona with fertility issues. Because I was paying her, I knew she was there purely to help me and to work out what I needed to get through treatment.

The treatment went well and, incredibly, it worked first time. Said and I were so excited. When I was seven weeks pregnant, a blood test showed that my levels of beta hCG had started to fall, and the doctors advised me to have IVIg (intravenous immunoglobulin), as they thought an immune problem might be stopping implantation and causing the drop. It was a relief to see a heartbeat on the scan later that day.

Then, at a scan a week later, the heartbeat wasn't there any more. I was on my own when I found out, as Said was working. It was awful. Said told me later that when I called, his legs went weak and he very nearly collapsed.

The miscarriage scarred both of us. I went into hospital on a holy day, Eid, to have the operation to remove the pregnancy. I didn't want to wait for my body to expel it naturally: I'd seen a friend go through waiting for that to happen, and it had been horrendous for her. I felt I had to get the operation over with, and move on quickly to let my body heal.

Friends were shocked by the miscarriage, and didn't know what to say. I remember one friend saying, 'Don't worry, you can try again'. But we'd already spent £5000, and there was no guarantee that I'd get pregnant again. It sounds awful, but I felt that even anyone who'd had a miscarriage after getting pregnant naturally wouldn't understand. It had been such a long road to get pregnant in the first place.

A few weeks later, my sister gave birth to her second child. I spiralled into emotional chaos, completely floored. On top of all that, at work, I was called into a management meeting and told that the funding for the parenting support service wasn't going to continue, and that I'd have to tell three people in my team that they would no longer have jobs. At that point, I broke down and cried, which I'd never done before at work. My managers looked shocked. I could have coped with just one thing, but I was overwhelmed by what seemed like loss after loss.

I'd become sensitised to pregnant women and small babies, and every time I saw either I broke down. But as I wound down the service, I had to see patients to assess whether they needed to be referred on. And a lot of them were pregnant women and babies. So as a way of coping with that, I avoided seeing both in my personal life. Two or three of my friends were pregnant again, one of them for the sixth time. The only way I could deal with my raw emotions was to avoid situations that provoked them. I had to cut myself off and not attend christenings or parties. Some friends came to see me without their children, but I still felt very isolated.

The grief over the miscarriage was sometimes overwhelming. It frightened me just how dark my feelings were. I felt suicidal, though I wouldn't have acted on it. My GP suggested antidepressants but I didn't want to take them.

Three months later, Said and I started to discuss having treatment again. Because of the miscarriage, Said and I were, at that time, going through a kind of emotional separation, and he said he wouldn't come to the clinic with me. So I went to the appointments with a friend.

Anya normalised the fact that Said didn't seem to be on board with this treatment, and said he would be later on. She helped me to understand what he was going through, that he was still shell-shocked by the loss of the pregnancy. And she told me about a fertility website for men (mensfe.net), so he could look at it. Anya was right – Said did come round to the idea of us having IVF again; she understood that if I could get the support I needed from her and others, I was going to get through the treatment and be able to support Said through it too.

Looking at what had happened the previous cycle, the doctors said they suspected that it might have been immune problems that led to the miscarriage. I had tested borderline positive for lupus, an autoimmune disease, two years before, but I'd never made the link between that and not getting pregnant. When the clinic did the immune testing, lupus came up again, and the doctors told me this can stop the embryo from implanting. The treatment – though still experimental – is to have a course of a drug called HUMIRA. It's very expensive and extremely painful, as it has to be injected into your stomach muscles every two weeks for two months leading up to treatment. I cried after every single injection.

Two weeks before my 40th birthday, I'd finished the course of HUMIRA and was prepared for our next round of IVF. Then I had the blood test of my follicle-stimulating hormone (FSH) to see whether it was the right day to start treatment. A few hours later, I got a call from the clinic, to say my FSH level had gone up to 13, a sign that I was perimenopausal. It had never been high before, but the ARGC won't treat you on the cycles where your FSH is above 10. When I hung up the phone, I sobbed and sobbed. There was a chance that in a month or two the level would come down again, but there was no guarantee. And if it didn't, our next option would be egg donation. Both Said and I knew that was an absolute no-no, for religious reasons, but also for personal ones too.

For the next two weeks, I tried to pretend I was fine and carry on as normal. I'd organised a party of 10 of my closest female friends to go to lunch at Kensington Roof Gardens on my birthday, and for me to go out with Said in the evening. I couldn't handle a big party, so I downgraded the celebration to a dinner in the local Italian. My sisters arrived to stay with me before my birthday and, finally, I fell apart. I couldn't even face the low-key dinner. I felt so ashamed and so sad that I might never get pregnant. My sisters rang my friends to cancel.

That was both my and Said's lowest point. I saw Anya every week. I felt completely overwhelmed, so she made me look back at my fertility journey, and realise how far I'd come. The image she used was of climbing Everest in small steps. Every session, she would break things down into my steps for that day or week, so I'd concentrate on the next blood test, rather than the possible result.

Anya also helped by focusing on the practical – like looking online for a diet that helps with fertility. I showed it to Said, and he started making me really healthy fresh food. I began taking a supergreen supplement, with algae and wheatgrass, which some nutritionists think can help. And I found an excellent shiatsu practitioner, who pummelled out my stress in a weekly massage. With Anya, I had a private place where I could be vulnerable, but she'd always give me a goal at the end of every session.

When I had my next blood test, to see if my FSH was low enough to start, it was back down to nine. I started IVF that day. At the end of two weeks, I produced 10 follicles, then had three embryos put back in. I got pregnant again. This time, it was hard to feel confident that the pregnancy would last, especially as I bled at eight weeks. It wasn't until the pregnancy started to show that Said would even talk about it. Then I bled at 15 weeks. And, at 26 weeks, I was hospitalised when doctors thought I was losing the baby.

Every time I had a scan, Said couldn't bear to come in with me. Instead, he'd sit outside the door, listen to what the sonographer was saying, and to my breathing. He'd hear the silence as I held my breath when the probe was first put on my stomach. And he said he knew everything was ok when he heard me breathe out again.

Even at the end, Said refused to come to the delivery, so my mum was with me when Sumaya was born by C-section. But he did come in after she was born, and the nurse handed her to him. Afterwards, he told me that he was uncertain at first, as he'd read horror stories about sperm and eggs being mixed up at clinics, but when he saw Sumaya, he knew she was his. She looks so like him. Then he followed the Muslim tradition of the father whispering particular words of the

Qu'ran into the newborn's ears. He said it was an amazing moment.

It's so painful when you're going through infertility. But now Sumaya is eight months old, I feel I've got to a place where I can look back on what happened. I'm delighted to have a daughter. But I still feel sad and cheated that I didn't experience falling pregnant naturally. Even now, when people talk about getting pregnant easily or by accident, it bites into the wound caused by infertility. It would be amazing to pee on a stick, get a positive result and not even have tried.

One of my sisters is pregnant with her fourth child. I always thought I'd have four or five children and, even after having Sumaya, I felt a stab of jealousy and hurt hearing she was pregnant. I know I have my happy ending, but there's still a feeling of loss. I wish Sumaya could have siblings, but I've realised I will probably never hold another baby of my own again.

Q: WHO SUPPORTED YOU DURING TREATMENT?

When we first had problems getting pregnant, I felt very lonely. I didn't want to go online for support – I was terrified that I'd buddy up with someone, then she'd get pregnant, and that would be too much for me.

Anya, my fertility coach, advised me to build up a support network. My network was small, but it worked: one friend, the one who'd had twins through IVF at the same clinic as me, was the person who accompanied me to appointments; another, who is really into art and culture, would organise nice outings to the opera and theatre; a third, a very devout Muslim, prayed for me, and she would give me *hadith*, inspirational teachings, from the Qu'ran. (After the miscarriage, she told me that according to Islam, if you lose a child, that child goes ahead of you to the gates of heaven, and waits for you to come there. And you hold their hand to bring them into heaven. Images like that kept me going.)

Q: WHY DID YOU CHOOSE COACHING?

I could have chosen to have the sort of therapy I'd had when I was doing my professional training, but it went too deep. Or I could have had counselling, which is a useful place to dump feelings but, for me at the time, it didn't provide the practical help I needed. I knew I wanted something less in-depth than therapy, someone who could work with me in a targeted, goal-focused way, and coaching fitted the bill.

Q: HOW DO YOU KNOW WHEN YOU'VE FOUND THE RIGHT 'THERAPIST'?

It's down to the strength of the therapeutic relationship. If the relationship isn't right, it won't work. When you're under a great deal of stress and looking for a caregiver, the theory is that you're revisiting your earliest caregiver relationship – that of the mother and baby. You're looking for someone with natural warmth, an ability to 'get' you and what you're feeling, and an emotional robustness, so you know he or she is secure enough to cope with your emotional stress. That last point was important for me – my emotions can be very overwhelming, but Anya was able to deal with them.

Q: HOW DID COACHING HELP YOU?

I'd thought that all couples went through IVF together. My belief that you're supposed to be totally in synch as a couple would have been really corrosive if Anya hadn't explained that it's not true.

Men don't have the same support systems as women, so their partners are their main support. Although we didn't have coaching together, it put me in a better position to help Said.

It also helped me to cope with strong emotions. There was envy, which I'd never felt before. And anger – at times, I felt extreme anger towards women who could become pregnant easily. Those feelings have stuck with me and I know they have deepened my professional work.

• • • • • • • • •

Whatever help you think you need, make sure you get it, whether it's counselling, therapy or coaching. Coaching is different from counselling, in that it's about developing concrete strategies for coping. 'Counsellors think it works best when offered alongside counselling,' says Mollie Graneek.

Fertility coach, Anya Sizer, has written a practical book, *Fertile Thinking* (Infinite Ideas), to help you through the process of IVF. And there's a more holistic approach, based on relaxation techniques in *Conquering Infertility: Dr. Alice Domar's Mind/Body Guide to Enhancing Fertility and Coping with Infertility* (Penguin Books). Dr Domar is an American health psychologist and creator of the hugely successful Mind/Body programmes (in the UK, they are run at the London Bridge Fertility, Gynaecology and Genetics Centre – thebridgecentre.co.uk). A colleague who did the course said that it was incredible, and helped her to get through IVF with a lot less stress than previously.

Do ask your GP to refer you for counselling, so you can get it free, though there's often a waiting list. At some clinics, a session of counselling is included in a cycle, others just recommend counsellors. To find a counsellor with expertise in fertility issues, go to the British Infertility Counselling Association website (bica.net).

My friends and family got me through

• • • • • • • • • • • •

T wo of the questions I heard the most during the research for this book were, who should you tell about fertility problems and what should you say when you do? Do you keep the fact you're having IVF between the two of you, so that if the treatment doesn't work, you don't have explain what's happened multiple times? Or do you share what's going on, so you feel supported?

'Family members who you've always been close to, or friends you love to bits aren't always as helpful as you'd expect because IVF is such a unique and specific situation,' says fertility coach, Anya Sizer. 'They probably won't understand the specifics of, for example, FSH levels, drug regimes and embryo development that you've had to learn.'

Now IVF is more mainstream than it used to be, it is easier to talk about. But the flip side is that because it's in the news so much, everyone's suddenly a fertility expert. And people often say exactly the wrong thing. 'It's just a ball of cells at that stage,' after a failed cycle, for example or, my favourite after my miscarriage: 'At least you know you can get pregnant.'

Anya's advice to anyone going through IVF is to create a support network. And to tell those people exactly what you need when you need it, whether it's more space, practical help or just a hug. 'What tends to happen during IVF number one is that the couple find most of the support from each other,' says Anya. 'If it doesn't work, the woman then looks externally for support, whether it's from friends, family or online. This, it's good to realise, is healthy and normal, not a sign of something going wrong in the relationship.'

In online fertility forums, at least everyone knows what you're going through and is as obsessed as you about treatment details. And you can be 100 per cent honest about your emotions too. 'Do handle the internet slightly wisely though,' says Anya. 'There's a lot of medical information online written by patients, which can be confusing; and some of it is just plain wrong.'

Sizer also advises that you prepare for tough real-life situations. For example, have someone on speed dial for when a colleague announces her pregnancy, or rehearse something to say when you're cornered at a family wedding by a kindly relative who tells you not to leave having children too late. It's worth reading the bloggers who say exactly what you're thinking and help you laugh at your situation, especially 999reasonstolaugh.com by 'Infertile Naomi'. My favourite from her? 'You know you're infertile when … Everyone at the fertility clinic knows your name, including the nurses and secretary. It's like an episode of *Cheers*, just without the bar and unlimited alcohol.'

● ● ● ● ● ● ● ● ●

Before Karen, 31, an administration assistant from Nottinghamshire, had IVF treatment, she created a network of support.

I've never met my best friend Kelly, even though we've been emailing each other regularly for three years. We talk on the phone nearly every day, and send each other photos of our children, as well as birthday and Christmas presents. We've tried to arrange days out together, but now we've both got twins and Kelly is about to have her third baby, I'm not sure when it'll happen.

Kelly and I first met online, on the Fertility Friends website, before either of us had started IVF. When she posted on the site for the first time, her story sounded so like mine that I sent her a personal message. It turned out we had an awful lot in common: we'd both been with our partners since we were teenagers, we'd both been trying for babies for eight years and we both had 'unexplained' infertility. Since then, we've been through every step of the fertility journey together: tests, IVF, the two-week wait, twin pregnancies.

Kelly probably knows more about me than any of my other friends. Right from our first conversation, Kelly was someone I knew would understand exactly what I was going through with infertility and who would always be there for me. She knew she could call me at any time, too.

By the time I was 22, Mark and I had decided to start a family. I assumed it would just happen for us. I'm from a big family – my mum is one of 13 – so there always seemed to be someone in the family having a baby. No one I knew had ever had any trouble conceiving before.

After we'd tried for a year, we thought we should get checked out. It took the best part of another year to have all the fertility tests we needed, waiting for appointments, which was a frustrating time. It turned out that Mark's sperm was fine, my hormones were fine and my tubes weren't blocked. My periods had always been heavy and very painful, so I had a laparoscopy; I think the surgeon was expecting to find a cyst, fibroid or even endometriosis, but there was only one tiny cyst on one of my ovaries, which he removed.

That left us with a diagnosis of 'unexplained' infertility. My consultant told me my weight could be the issue, and that I needed to get my BMI down to 25. I'm quite short – five foot one – and, at the time, I weighed nearly 12 stone, so my BMI was 31. I went all out to lose weight: I exercised every day on our ski machine at home, did sit-ups and ate really well.

Eight months later, we went back. I'd lost six pounds and asked to be put on the waiting list for IVF, but the consultant said I needed to lose more weight first. I was so disappointed. It felt as if I wasn't a priority because I was only 23. I couldn't go back to see that consultant again because I couldn't talk to her – she made me feel so uncomfortable. We felt as though we'd hit a wall with the NHS, that we wouldn't get any more help from them. So we thought we'd try again to get pregnant naturally.

We changed what we ate, so we were eating home-cooked organic food and we cut out all processed foods, takeaways and fizzy pop. I switched to decaffeinated tea and coffee and started taking a fertility supplement. I made poor Mark eat packs and packs of Brazil nuts, as they contain a lot of selenium, a mineral that's good for sperm quality. We followed all the natural fertility advice we could find. I even tried staying in bed with my legs up after sex.

When, after another year, it still hadn't worked, we thought it might be because we were getting so stressed about doing everything right. We weren't enjoying life, and decided that if we just relaxed a bit, I might get pregnant. So for a few years, we put the whole issue of children on the back burner.

But that didn't stop members of the family asking us when we were planning to have children. Their questions made a hard situation worse, as it made me feel that I was letting them down too. Mark was a big support: we always told each other that if we couldn't have children, we'd still be happy together.

Just before my 28th birthday, I told Mark that if we were going to give IVF a go, I wanted to do it before I was 30. Luckily, we had enough money to go privately.

Once I've decided to do something, I like to get going, so we found a clinic close to us, booked a consultation and both of us had tests. Everything looked fine: my hormones were at the right level and Mark's sperm was good quality. An internal scan revealed that my antral follicle count (AFC) was good too. The AFC is the number of follicles that you start growing each month, and it's an indication of the number of follicles that will grow during IVF. We were ready to go.

The nurses described our cycle as 'textbook'. Everything went well, from down-regulation to the steady growth of my follicles and the thickening of the lining of my womb. In the end, I had 10 eggs collected and nine of them fertilised. On day three, I had two embryos put back: one had divided to six cells, and one had grown to eight cells. The other seven embryos had stopped growing that morning, but we didn't want them to go to waste, so we signed them over to research.

Mark was in the room, holding my hand tightly during the transfer. The embryologist put the pictures of the embryos up on the screen before they went in. Each just looked like a brown circle, but it was breathtaking to see something that could have the potential to become a human being.

The two-week wait was an exciting time. I felt as if I was pregnant for the very first time in my life. I'd never even had a pregnancy scare before or been a single day late for my period. Mark wouldn't let me do anything at all; he made me just lie down at home.

Then, eight days later, I started bleeding. At first, it was a little bit of blood. But by the end of the day, it was a full-on period, with my usual cramping pains. We were both distraught. I went to the loo in the bathroom, and I shouted for Mark to come, saying, 'I'm really bleeding, now. I think it's over.' I was crying; Mark hugged me and said we'd try again, that it wasn't the end of the world.

I don't know what I would have done without Kelly. When I told her what had happened, she was very upset and we both had a cry. She was so supportive and helped turn my thinking around until I was positive. She sent me a lovely card to say she was thinking about me, and that she knew one day I'd be a mummy, and a great one.

The girls on Fertility Friends were great too, because they understood exactly what I was going through. I knew they weren't going to judge me, and the fact they didn't know me personally was a good thing, so I could share every detail without ever feeling embarrassed.

For the next few days, I was very quiet and withdrawn. Mark knows that if I'm being quiet, and I don't want to talk about something, it's better to leave me alone until I'm ready. I deal better with things by processing them on my own. At first, I blamed myself because the doctors had done everything to help me get pregnant, but I just couldn't hold on to it. Had I rested enough or too much? Had I eaten the wrong things? After some soul-searching, I came to the conclusion that I hadn't done anything wrong, that it was just one of those things.

But every time I went to the bathroom, I was reminded of what had happened; I wasn't sure I could go through IVF again – all the injections and scans and procedures. And, most of all, the hope; because everything had seemed to go so well, it was a huge blow. We were given a 67 per cent chance of it working at my age, so I think we'd got over-confident. To get so close to having what we'd always wanted was terrible; it felt as if it had been snatched away.

The official pregnancy test came back negative, as we'd expected. We discussed trying again straight away, which I wanted to do. I thought if I waited, I was in danger of changing my mind. At my follow-up consultation at the clinic, the consultant suggested a three-month break, but when I insisted, he agreed there was no reason I couldn't start immediately.

I was much more relaxed for the next cycle. I decided not to have acupuncture – it had cost £900 – and to be more laid back about what we were eating too. I realised I'd tried to do too much differently during our first cycle, including drinking pints and pints of milk, which I hate. This time, I had coffee, if only a cup in the morning, and if I wanted a fizzy drink, I had one.

Luckily, I had an understanding boss and my job was flexitime, so it wasn't too hard getting to appointments. Theresa, Mark's sister, very sweetly came with me to the clinic when Mark couldn't, and I always had the Fertility Friends girls to chat to online when I was feeling stressed.

The treatment went well again: I grew 15 follicles, my lining was even thicker, and, in the end, I had 10 eggs which all fertilised. We had a day-three transfer again and, this time, both embryos were eight cells. This was slightly better than before, although they weren't such good quality. Embryos are graded according to how 'fragmented' they are. The more whole and tidy the embryo looks, the better it is. On the first cycle, the embryos were grade two, and this time they were grade two/three.

Every day of the two-week wait I expected to get my period, but it didn't come. The night before test day, Mark and I were discussing what time to wake up, and I said, 'I can't do the test, you'll have to'. We decided to set the alarm for 4.30 a.m., that I'd wee in a plastic pot, then Mark would go into the bathroom to put the stick in. That was the first time in eight and a half years of trying that we'd got to the stage of doing a pregnancy test. I went for a pee, gave him the pot and the test and got back under the covers. A couple of minutes later, Mark came to the bedroom door. I couldn't tell the result from his face, but he said, 'What does two lines mean?' I said, 'Mark, don't joke about this.' I got out of bed, read the instructions as fast as I could and saw that two lines meant it was positive. We looked at each other, burst out crying, then cuddled and kissed for ages.

I had bought some more tests and, over the next few hours, did seven of them, just to check the result. At 7 a.m., we called our parents, then Theresa, who was so thrilled for us that she cried. When I rang Kelly, she screamed down the phone and she cried too. Then I posted our great news online, and got loads more congratulations.

I went to work, even though I'd had no sleep and was in a world of my own. It was early, and the only other person who was in was a colleague who'd been supportive all the way through my treatment. She had children, and understood why I wanted a family. When I sat down at my desk, I burst into tears. She asked me what was wrong, and I told her my news; she gave me a hug and said how happy she was for us. I explained that I wasn't going to tell anyone else for a few days, as I needed time for it to sink in.

The next four weeks, waiting for my first scan at eight weeks, went very slowly. I was trying to keep positive – we'd got this far – and I wanted to enjoy being pregnant, but I was so frightened it would be taken away from me. The day before the scan, I started feeling sick, and I put it down to nerves. I was actually sick the morning of the scan, but, again, I thought it was because it was such a big day.

Everyone at the clinic congratulated me when I arrived; it's such a small clinic that I'd got to know all the staff. The consultant I'd had throughout did the scan, which was reassuring. His first words were, 'Look, here's the heartbeat,' and I felt a whoosh of relief in my stomach. Then he went quiet, and I thought something was wrong. I didn't move a muscle. Then he said, 'And here's another one. Congratulations, you're having twins.'

Mark and I just looked at each other, saying nothing. It had been amazing to be told we were having one baby, but having two was a miracle. When I got dressed, we went to the car to drive home. But neither of us could move for a good half an hour, or say anything. We just sat there.

We knew that the whole family was on tenterhooks, waiting for us to call with the scan result, but we couldn't. When I eventually managed to call and say the words, 'Everything's fine, and we're having twins,' for the first time, it was lovely. They were all so happy, I couldn't help but get emotional again. I still felt sick, and Mark said it was probably shock, but, in fact, I suffered terribly with morning sickness from then on.

It wasn't until our 20-week scan that I felt safely pregnant, which is also when we discovered we were having a boy and a girl. When my sickness finally stopped, when I was 24 weeks pregnant, I started shopping, buying blue and pink, and making the most of feeling better. I also felt more confident because I knew that for every week past 24, the babies would have a better chance of survival.

I felt mostly well, though I was diagnosed with gestational diabetes, so I had to inject myself with insulin in the thigh every day. But the needles didn't faze me after all those weeks of IVF injections.

As my due date got closer, I had to give up work because I was so big, I couldn't fit behind my steering wheel. By 37 weeks, I was begging to be induced, I was so enormous. The babies were already a healthy size, so I was finally induced at 37 weeks and 3 days. I was in labour for 19 hours. They had to make a little cut to help Lexi out, who was 5lb 4oz. Mitchell was 6lb 8oz and breech, so they pulled him out by his feet and, sadly, fractured a bone in his arm in the process. But luckily, neither twin needed to go into special care, and I only spent four days in hospital. It was a lovely end to years of infertility, and it was also an amazing beginning to our family life.

Q: WHO WAS YOUR SUPPORT GROUP DURING IVF?

I knew I needed different kinds of support during treatment. I had Mark, of course, who made sure he was a big part of the treatments, getting my injections ready for me, and coming to every appointment he could. It's easy for women to feel as if they're doing absolutely everything, and their partner is doing nothing, but that wasn't true for us.

I also think it's important to have someone to rely on who's not your partner. Otherwise, fertility would have been all Mark and I ever talked about, and we would have driven each other mad. Mark had a close friend who he could confide in. And I had Mark's sister Theresa who, although she's never been through infertility, is like a little sister to me. She came to appointments when Mark couldn't, and was always there to give me a hug when I needed one.

Then I had the girls on Fertility Friends, in particular Kelly, who was there for me every day of my treatment, as I was for her when she went through IVF a few months after me. Anyone who's been through infertility understands not only the practical side, but also the overwhelming emotions and the ups and downs. Every time I went on to Fertility Friends, I knew I'd find someone who was willing to help or share her experience. It's a great community.

We were very selective about who else we told, in 'real life', about having treatment, mainly because we didn't want to have to explain if it wasn't successful. We only told our immediate family – parents, brothers and sisters. I was happy for my mum to tell her sister too: she needed someone to support her, especially when she was so upset after the first treatment didn't work. The second time, we did tell more friends and family, but the date we gave them for the pregnancy test was two days after it was actually scheduled. I thought that would give me time to get my head around the result, whatever it was.

Q: WHAT'S THE BEST AGE TO HAVE IVF?

Don't think you're too young to have treatment. Even in our early 20s, we needed help but we were put off asking for it. I don't think the doctors take you so seriously when you're younger. But it's better to try when you're younger if you can, as your chances are so much better.

Q: HOW SHOULD YOU REACT WHEN FRIENDS OR FAMILY GIVE UNWANTED ADVICE?

Take anyone's advice with a pinch of salt. If they're not a doctor or nurse, or haven't had fertility issues, they probably know less than you do. I can't count the number of times that people told me to put my legs up after sex, but not everyone who gets pregnant has done that. And there were all those times in eight years that people – usually those who'd got pregnant easily – said, 'Relax, don't get stressed, and it'll happen'.

If you're feeling awkward, and it's someone you know well, you could say, 'Please don't tell me what to do, as you've never had this problem'. If you don't know the person so well, it's better to humour them, rather than get into a debate. I used to try and say something like, 'Yes, we'll definitely try that', then change the subject.

Q: WHAT'S THE BEST WAY TO KEEP YOUR RELATIONSHIP SUPPORTIVE DURING IVF?

Talk to each other. It's important for the woman to talk about IVF, as it makes her partner feel needed, loved and involved and helps him to understand what she's going through. There's not much for the man to do during IVF, so he can easily feel like a spare part.

Although IVF is tough on both of you, mentally and emotionally, try to do things together in your relationship that you always liked, so there's some kind of normality. For example, we carried on going out for meals and walking the dogs together. In the end, IVF made us stronger, as it made me appreciate how Mark makes everything seem possible. It made me love him more.

• • • • • • • • •

With advice from fertility coach, Anya Sizer, I created my own support team for my last two cycles. I was lucky enough to see acupuncturist, Emma Cannon, for treatments and a chat and fertility expert Zita West, who talked me through practical decisions. Then there were the five friends, two colleagues and Mum, who sent me daily texts and emails, and who acted as my cheerleaders, whatever the latest report from the clinic. Not forgetting the women on the #infertility and #ivf groups on Twitter, where I met some international cycle buddies. And my husband, of course, who hated coming to appointments so much that instead, he drove me there, then went home and cooked delicious and nutritious food for me.

Most people were kind and tried to be sensitive, but there were also those who didn't really understand why I was having IVF. For example, one family member questioned whether I should have it: 'Do you want children that much?'

Almost all the women I spoke to for the book said they had lost some friendships over having fertility problems. Writer Carrie Friedman has written a brilliant piece for the *LA Times* on what not to say to someone who's having fertility treatment (find it at www.latimes.com/health/la-he-my-turn-infertility-20110425,0,470341.story). And there's a very funny blog called Infertility Etiquette at www.fertilityauthority.com/blogger/jay-bronte/2011/04/04/infertility-etiquette. 'Understand if you're pregnant and I don't talk to you for a while, it's nothing personal, I just hate your uterus,' says its author Jay Bronte. And she has some more serious advice too: 'Please no anecdotes and no advice ... Please don't suggest using donor sperm or donor eggs ... If you have children or are pregnant, please don't talk about the downside ... Please don't mention celebrities who went through infertility.' Print out her list of things that can be unintentionally hurtful when dealing with infertility and give them out to friends and family.

My experience
of miscarriage

• • • • • • • • • • • •

I s miscarriage worse after IVF? The accepted professional view is that pretty much all pregnancy loss, whenever it happens, should be treated equally. 'You can't
compare one person's loss to another's. Nor can you compare
miscarriage after IVF to other miscarriage, because everyone
is different. Just because someone else has a stillbirth,
doesn't make your pain any less,' says M, a counsellor at
CARE Fertility.

A friend, who has managed teams of women for 20 years,
admits she judges friends' and employees' miscarriages on a
sliding scale: that is, how many you have had, if you have
children, how far along you were, how hard it was to get
pregnant and how hard it might be to get pregnant again. In
some ways, I can understand her view.

I'm in no way implying that miscarriage after natural
conception isn't equally painful, especially for those women
who have more than one miscarriage. But there is something
particularly cruel about miscarriage after infertility. In my

case, I was one day shy of 16 weeks pregnant when I lost the pregnancy. I felt I'd been preparing for IVF, eating and drinking like a pregnant woman, praying to be pregnant, doing IVF and actually being pregnant for over a year.

'Miscarriage is always a devastating experience, but it's made more painful by the fact that couples doing IVF often cannot try naturally for another pregnancy,' says M. 'They have to go through more treatment, with no guarantee of success at the end of it.'

But she adds, after miscarriage everyone – no matter how they conceived – has to go through a process of grieving for the loss of the child they had been expecting. 'Most medical professionals now recognise the profound emotional effect that miscarriage has on both a woman and her partner.'

The grieving, says M, is similar to any other kind of loss, in all its confusion of feelings. 'There's a sense of shock and/or disbelief. And there's a searching: why did this happen? You might be angry, and blame someone: whether that's the doctors or clinic staff, or even the bus driver who drove too fast over bumps. Or yourself. You may think: should I have taken more notice of a certain symptom? Or seen a doctor earlier? You may have feelings of hopelessness or become depressed. And, if you've had a termination earlier in your life, you might feel you're being punished.'

What helps is talking – to friends, family and, in particular, to a counsellor or professional. 'Talking – and crying – can help with the healing process of grief. Seeing a professional counsellor can also help to work through the confusion of painful feelings.' The idea is that by talking through what's happened to you, you can come to some kind of resolution: whether you can bear to have IVF again, or not.

● ● ● ● ● ● ● ●

Brigid, 41, a journalist from London, thought that once she'd got through IVF, nothing else could go wrong.

I stared at the faint cross on the pregnancy test, my brain not believing what my eyes could see. What a place to find out I was pregnant. I was at the Fertility Show in London, in some institutional Formica-lined loos, in the bowels of the Olympia conference centre. I found I couldn't speak or even dial a number on my phone, so I just kept staring at the faint cross on the stick, and smiling, but also crying, with relief and happiness.

I'd been so sure that the IVF treatment hadn't worked this time. And I wasn't supposed to be testing – it was three days before my proper pregnancy blood test was due. But after listening to three hours of talks that morning by doctors on the ins and outs of IVF, I hadn't been able to resist going into a chemist at lunchtime and buying a pack of tests.

Walking out of the loos, the women coming in probably thought I was crying because I wasn't pregnant, when the opposite was true. In the crowded exhibition hall upstairs, the first person I bumped into was Zita West, the fertility expert who'd helped me decide that I would try again for this last time. 'Oh my God, Zita, I'm pregnant,' I blurted, trying to keep my voice down, knowing I was surrounded by women who wanted to be. She hugged me, congratulated me, hugged me again and told me to go and sit down, take a breath.

I called Adam, my husband, who was delighted. 'I knew you could do it,' he said. I imagined our perfect family; our gorgeous three-year-old, Patrick, also an IVF baby, and a little sibling – boy or girl? – who would make us the luckiest parents in London. My chances of success, at 41, were 12.5

per cent, looking at the national figures. At my clinic, the ARGC in London, they were 31.5 per cent.

After a successful first cycle – that was Patrick – one failed frozen cycle and a failed fresh cycle, the last one just nine months before, I had beaten the odds, it seemed. I sat through a presentation by Mr Mohamed Taranissi, medical director of the ARGC, smiling inanely at him, not really taking in the discussions on the platform. In my brain, all I could hear was, I'm pregnant! I'm pregnant! I'm pregnant!

At home, Adam and I hugged and I cried again. I was cautiously optimistic about this baby; my previous pregnancy with Patrick, nearly four years before, had been textbook. This time though, after blood tests, I was put on a lot more drugs: clexane to thin my blood, baby aspirin to do the same, the steroid prednisolone, as my tests had shown slightly raised natural-killer cell levels (I wasn't sure I believed in NK cells, but I thought I should do whatever the doctors said – it had worked last time). And there was the nightly ordeal of my progesterone injection, which went deep into the muscle of my bottom via a needle big enough to use on a horse.

It felt very different, being pregnant at 41 to doing it at 36. I felt 20 years more tired, not just four. And, from five weeks onwards, I was nauseous and drained all day. What saved me was sugar: banana smoothies, pints of Ribena and juice and hot chocolate. A combination of the IVF drugs, the steroids, my sugar intake and the fact it was my second pregnancy meant I started to show early, around eight weeks.

Both Adam and I were so looking forward to the baby, though I refused to talk about it until after the 12-week scan. It seemed like too much of a miracle. Having had three embryos put back, I was dreading the fact that it could so easily be twins, especially given that my beta hCG pregnancy hormone levels were very high. I thought I might prefer a girl, and I'd call her Hero. If it was a boy, I was torn between

Joseph and Sidney. Looking back, I can't believe I cared about anything other than having a healthy baby.

Because it was New Year, the whole family came to the 12-week scan: my husband, Patrick and me. We saw the baby: it looked like a boy to me: a big head, big nose, nothing like Patrick's more delicate features in his 12-week scan picture. He (or she) was moving so much, the doctor couldn't get the final delicate heart calculation for 10 minutes. Patrick got impatient in the meantime and started jumping around, moving chairs. Finally, the doctor managed to get the reading, and worked out our odds of the baby having Down's syndrome or another genetic abnormality. It was one in 2000, incredibly low for my age. We were lucky yet again. We had a family hug, then went for a posh burger. I ate chips and laughed a lot, relieved.

Announcing the pregnancy in the New Year at work was lovely, with lots of congratulations. Most people knew how much we had put into this pregnancy, how long we had waited. My editor hugged me, said, 'Congratulations! You deserve it,' and tweeted my news. I was officially pregnant, at last.

I did start to feel better, less tired, at 14 weeks, but only for a week. I thought I was overtired or had developed early 'pregnancy brain', as I couldn't think straight. I had a sore on my hand that wouldn't heal and sores at the corners of my mouth too. Then, for a few nights I was up with a full bladder, trying to pee and not being able to. Three days later, on a Saturday, I started to bleed. Just a little, but red blood – the type the books always say is not a good sign. And I had a strange feeling, as if my cervix was dropping down. So off we went to St Mary's A & E department. The GP there did a urine test, took my blood pressure and pulse and sent me up to see the gynaecologist on duty.

In the emergency gynaecology room, I was scanned. A huge relief: the baby was still wriggling away. By then, the bleeding had stopped. I didn't feel well – I told the gynaecologist about not being able to pee sometimes. But the A&E GP had said that the dipstick had showed no signs of infection, and when the gynaecologist examined me internally she said everything looked fine, that my cervix was closed. She scanned me before and after I peed, and said I wasn't emptying my bladder. She told me I should make sure I emptied my bladder at night, in case it caused an infection. She also said that bleeding can be a sign that a pregnancy is ending, or it can be nothing, and that there wasn't much any doctor could do to change that.

So I put all my symptoms down to pregnancy – the tiredness, the sores, my bladder, not being able to concentrate and, on Monday at work, feeling exhausted and unable to cope.

Three days later, I woke up early, bleeding again. I had a throbbing pain in my lower back and couldn't get comfortable in bed. I called a cab to go to the hospital. I think on some level I knew what was about to happen, but the doctor had said I was fine, so I hung on to that. Sitting in my kitchen, waiting for the cab, I whispered to the baby, 'Don't come now, it's too early'.

The rush-hour traffic was terrible on the way to the hospital, and the pain was getting worse. The taxi driver wouldn't take any money, bless him. At the antenatal clinic, the receptionist sent me straight to the emergency gynaecology unit. That meant more waiting – ironically, at the end of the corridor where I'd sat for so many hours in the past waiting for fertility appointments and investigations. My chair was opposite the receptionist's desk. Every so often, I'd double up in pain and she, looking embarrassed, would stare at her screen.

I went in to be examined. Again, the scan looked fine and the baby was wriggling even more. I thought the doctor seemed quite dismissive at first. I told her I had cramping pains, and when she examined me, she said I was most probably experiencing the usual growing pains of pregnancy. Then she looked at my notes from the previous week on the computer screen, and saw that the results of my urine test had showed I did have a urine infection; it seemed to me that was when she started to take me seriously. I began to get upset: why hadn't anyone contacted me about those results? The hospital? Or my GP? 'Yes,' said the doctor, 'it looks as if there's been a breakdown in communication.'

I started to feel sick, and the nurse brought me one of those cardboard hospital bowls. Kneeling on the floor, I vomited and filled it. When the nurse took my temperature, it was high and my pulse was fast. The doctor said they would admit me to the gynaecology ward to give me antibiotics. She said my urinary infection had probably turned into a renal infection, as I seemed 'quite unwell'. I refused an anti-sickness injection – I didn't want to hurt the baby.

The next five hours are a blur: lying on the examination bed in the scanning room; waiting to be admitted. I tried to get comfortable, to stop the pain that was now coming in waves. I'd forgotten my mobile, so asked to use the telephone. I managed to remember Adam's number, and told him I was being admitted. He was at work and said he'd come afterwards, if he could find someone to look after Patrick.

I took some paracetamol, and fell into a doze. Then the pain woke me up. I should have known it was labour at that point, but I didn't want to believe it. And the doctor had told me the baby was fine. 'It's just a renal infection – I'll be ok once I get the drugs,' I kept telling myself.

Although I was by then delirious, I could hear what was happening at the desk outside the office. First, it sounded as if there were no beds on the gynaecology ward, then, a few hours later, there were beds. The nurse came in to tell me I'd be moved soon, and gave me more painkillers. She said, 'Yes, renal infections can be very painful'.

No porter arrived to move me and, by this time, the pain was so bad that I had to stand up when the waves came, and bend over, holding on to the bed. A porter finally appeared, but without a wheelchair. I heard them send him away. He didn't come back. I watched the hands on the clock on the wall go round.

Finally, a porter came, but still no wheelchair. And the lift was being serviced. He left me sitting at the top of the stairs, and went down to the bottom of six flights to bring up a stair-lift. Slowly. Very slowly. I couldn't wait any longer and started to walk down the stairs. A nurse took my arm. Every so often, I had to stop because the pain was so bad.

At the bottom of the stairs, the porter went off to find a wheelchair. How hard would it have been to be prepared before, I thought? I started walking, crying hysterically by now. 'I just want the drugs,' I said. We were out in the open, between the hospital buildings. I felt horribly self-conscious, bent double with pain, scared I was going to vomit again.

Stopping by the lift, the nurse went off to find the porter, who was still looking for a wheelchair. I held on to the rail, having another wave of pain. Then the chair came, and I remember people moving out of the way so we could go into the lift. At times, I was in too much pain to sit down, so kept getting out of the chair. The nurse had to keep asking me to sit down.

We went to the same ward where I had seen the gynae-cologist the weekend before. The ward matron asked me which bed I wanted. Two beds free, I thought. And I'd been waiting five hours. Had there been one free all the time? 'I don't care – I just want the drugs to take the pain away,' I said. A nurse took me to the bed, gave me a gown to put on, but I was in so much agony, I couldn't even lie down. She told me afterwards that was when she knew what was about to happen.

When I managed to lie down, I curled up. Another nurse hooked me up to an IV drip, put the first dose of antibiotics into it and a fluid drip. I couldn't lie still. I felt wet suddenly, in my knickers. 'I'm not sure – it's not time, but I think my waters have broken,' I said.

The nurse told me they needed a urine sample, and I should come into the toilets, where they'd put a big cardboard bowl over the loo; I knew why, though I didn't want to believe it. The nurse held my hand as I sat on the loo. I felt a huge pain, and something slipped out of me. A white sac, the size of an apple, motionless, 'Oh, that wasn't supposed to happen,' I said. 'It's over, I can't believe it's over. That's so sad. That's the saddest thing.' More contractions, more stuff coming out. Then the placenta got stuck for what seemed like ages, more pain.

The nurse kept holding my hand, supporting me when I was sick again, putting my cardigan around my shoulders when I started shivering with the shock. Finally, after, it was all out, she led me back to the bed, and I lay down, still shivering.

I had more drips, more nurses. 'I'm sorry for your loss,' they said. A woman was shouting and cursing near by. It seemed utterly unreal: I curled up in a foetal position and cried. At the end of my bed, there was a room jutting into the ward, with walls made of white painted board. As I became more aware of what was going on, I realised the woman making all the noise was in labour in that room. She must have been in the transition phase, I thought, the part of labour where you get angry. 'Get off me,' she screamed repeatedly. 'I can't do it. Don't touch me.' Then, 'You're doing very well, Elizabeth,' from the midwife.

Why had they put me next to a woman giving birth? What horrible, thoughtless NHS planning had put me next to someone who was about to have the biggest joy of her life, I thought. Someone who'd be seeing her baby for the first time? The noise was constant and horrific. Gradually though, I realised that this wasn't an ordinary birth. The woman's screaming continued even after the last push of labour. 'Let me see the baby,' she said. 'Is it a boy or a girl? I'm psychic, I know it's a girl.' I don't know if the baby was dead or taken away – the nurses never told me anything about Elizabeth – but from what she was shouting, I knew the baby wasn't with her.

By now, I was plugged into a drip for hydration and one for antibiotics. I felt terrible – sick and shivery with shock. The nurses were kind; coming every so often to see how I was. I gave my number to a nurse to call Adam.

Late that afternoon, Adam arrived with Patrick. It was against the rules for the nurse to tell him what had happened on the phone, so he arrived expecting to see me pregnant, but having antibiotics for a renal infection. As Patrick cuddled me on the bed, I mouthed to him, 'I lost the baby'. His face looked so, so sad. Then I threw up again. Patrick was impressed; he'd never seen anyone else being sick before. It was all the water and orange juice I'd drunk since the miscarriage. 'Can I see it, Mummy?' he said. 'Oh! Yours is orange.'

Elizabeth was starting to wail again, her cries getting steadily louder, 'Give me my baby. I want my baby. Why won't you give me my baby?' and Patrick was beginning to get fidgety, trying to make the bed go up and down, running up the ward, so Adam took him home.

That night, Elizabeth continued shouting. She hadn't let the nurses take away the gas and air machine, and every hour or so she'd take a few huge mouthfuls and start shouting again. For a while it was, 'Daddy, come here. Help me.' And sometimes it was about God, or the baby. I hardly slept, just lay there, feeling sad, but also numb.

For the next two days, while I was in hospital, I think hardly ever saw the same doctor. The one who had been at the emergency gynaecology came and said she was sorry for my loss. Another doctor asked for my instructions about what to do with the body: did I want a funeral? No. Did I want a post-mortem on the body? I didn't think so. Did I want the placenta analysed? Yes.

The nurses were very good, especially those in charge. But seeing people I loved – Patrick, Adam, friends – was what mattered. The hospital food was indescribably bad – 'salmon bake' was a congealed, rancid mass of potatoes fried until deep brown in cheap oil and mixed with tinned salmon – but I didn't want to eat, so I didn't really care. One morning I ordered cornflakes, but couldn't eat them either; they'd been one of the things that had helped with my morning sickness.

Finally, after two nights, my fever was gone and my temperature was low enough for me to go home. It turned out that the miscarriage was caused by a bacteria called group A streptococcus. Things could have been worse. Strep A can go outside the womb, and cause a full-body infection that can even be fatal. It's one of the more unusual causes of miscarriage. 'Very unlucky,' said one doctor.

At home, I was in bed for a week. I was still on antibiotics – three different ones since they'd discovered the strep A – and feeling weak. I had lots of lovely messages, cards, flowers. I was pleased that most people had found out, so I didn't have to tell them. Every so often, I'd be overwhelmed by sadness, and cry for an hour. It was a sadness beyond anything I'd experienced. It was different from depression in its purity, but scarily similar in its desperation.

I was angry too: with the emergency gynaecologist for not being more thorough and not swabbing me to test for infection, with the hospital for not contacting me with my urine test results and with the second gynacologist for not realising

I was having contractions. I was angry with the series of hospital doctors, who I felt hadn't been able to answer most of my questions. I was angry with my midwife from when I had Patrick for not taking me on, so I'd had no one else to call about my symptoms. And with myself for not going to see my GP or even a private doctor. For not calling the IVF clinic. For not looking after the baby I'd been entrusted with properly. For letting him or her down. In my mind, I apologised to the baby, again and again.

Once I'd finished my three kinds of antibiotics, I began to feel a bit better, physically. Although I still felt fat and pregnant, which was a horrible contrast to my empty womb. My tummy and my breasts were swollen, a cruel reminder of what had happened every time I had a shower.

Seeing a counsellor did help, a little. She explained that all my feelings were normal, a process of bereavement that would go on for months, but would, she said, become easier with time. Being in a bubble at home was manageable; having breakfast with Patrick, going back to bed to sleep, then giving him a bedtime story after nursery. I felt as if I'd been wrapped in a warm blanket; Adam was very loving, fed me and looked after me. I cried for a while every day. Friends came over for cups of tea, making me laugh.

Sometimes, I'd think about killing myself, just to stop the horrible feelings. But I never ever would have done it: I knew life would be bearable in the future. Patrick saved me from my misery, really. Not only his hugs and kisses, but his constant questions about everything from the colour of eggs to where electricity comes from; the way he was working out how life worked made me smile. I knew how lucky I was to have him, how some women have miscarriage after miscarriage and little hope of ever having a child.

One day, a few days after I came home from hospital, Patrick wrapped up a cuddly lamb in a piece of paper, saying that he was too old for it, and wanted to give it to our baby when he came. I clenched my jaw, trying not to cry. 'The baby isn't coming now,' I said. 'Why, Mummy?' 'Because he was born too early. He was too small.' 'Why did he die, Mummy?' he said, coming straight to the point, as children do (we'd explained death when Bettler the rabbit had died in a fox attack a few weeks earlier). 'But why?' he asked again. 'I really did want us to have a baby. And why are you sad?' I was crying by then. I wanted to be honest with him but not scare him. 'Sometimes, babies are born too early, too small to live. And I'm sad because I really wanted the baby to come,' I said. 'But you make me happy, and I'm glad I've got you and Daddy because I love you both so much.'

That wasn't the last time Patrick talked about the baby. He must have known it was important; he must have seen how excited Adam and I were at the first scan, and heard my friends talking about the pregnancy, how amazing it was that I'd got pregnant. A few times, he asked me what the baby looked like when it came out. Tiny, like a little baby bird, I said. Was it moving when it came out of my tummy? No, I said. Did it know it was our baby? Was it too small even to know anything? Did it say, 'Mamma?' Where did it go after it died?

Back at work a few weeks later, I managed to keep it together at my desk, but found myself crying in the loos regularly. Everything set me off; an invitation to a press event on baby buggies, a news report about strep A killing new mothers. I couldn't look at dailymail.com because every day it announced another celebrity's pregnancy or admired her bump. Although, at the time, there was also news of Amanda Holden, who had lost her baby at almost seven months.

Adam and I finally had the huge row that had been brewing between us. I'd forgotten that he was sad too, so when I was feeling sad, I was sometimes cold to him. It was horrible to realise how wrapped up I'd been in myself. I brought up the subject of trying again. At first, I had been sure that I never wanted to do it again. Now I was back into writing the book, with all its stories of hope, I began to think that maybe, just maybe, we could be lucky. But Adam was certain. He didn't want to go through IVF again. 'We already have everything we need. Let's move on with life,' he said. He was being practical: we had already spent any money we had and borrowed the rest. I cried again at losing the chance of a second baby, at Patrick being a single child. But despite having a deep longing for a baby, I knew, logically, that Adam was right.

Now, two months on, I still cry when I'm alone. In my mind, I know I am lucky: a loving husband, an incredible, gorgeous son, a job that I love. Often, I feel guilty about being sad, as I know there are women who don't have a child, or who have even lost one. How can my pain compare to theirs? But if I don't cry and let the bad feelings out for a day or so, the guilt, anger, sadness, despair, they seep out and infect my day with paranoid anxiety: is Patrick's eye infection a deadly fungal one that will blind him? Is he going to fall and hit his head at nursery?

So I'm sad, but getting on with the usual stuff of life – even enjoying it sometimes. It's fun to be able to have a glass of wine, when I haven't drunk for so long. Or to take Patrick off to museums, or for a boat ride, or to a restaurant, without worrying about buggies and nap times and baby food. I know our family is going to be fine: smaller than we would have liked, but just the right size, all the same.

Q: WHAT WERE THE HARDEST PARTS?

The actual miscarriage – the physical feeling of the baby leaving my body is a memory that will never leave me. I am very grateful to the nurse who was with me at the time, for being so kind, and for not telling me what was going to happen before it happened.

For miscarriages after 12 weeks, the protocol is for the medical staff to ask you if you want to see the foetus, if you've had your miscarriage in hospital. That felt horrific to me at the time. I did see the foetus when it came out, but it was still in its white sac and I didn't want to remember him or her as dead. I can understand that for some people it would be important, particularly later on in a pregnancy.

The day after the miscarriage, a doctor went through the legal requirements: did I want a biopsy of the foetus or the placenta? Did I want a burial or for the foetus to be cremated? That was painful as it made it so real.

Telling Patrick, our four-year-old son, was hard, especially when he said, 'Mummy, but I wanted a baby'. I felt so guilty that I couldn't give him a brother or sister. And he still brings it up. Last week, he gave me a promotional postcard he'd picked up with a picture of a baby on the front. 'This is for you because your baby died,' he said.

And going back to work was tough, as for four weeks after the miscarriage I'd been protected at home. I had to face my friend who was pregnant in the office, babies in the street. It has got easier with time though.

Q: WHAT HELPED?

Because I was 16 weeks pregnant, everyone knew I was pregnant. So when people found out, they contacted me. It didn't matter what the message said, it was comforting thinking of those people thinking of me. Mothers, those who had had IVF and people who knew me and what I'd gone through to get pregnant said the right things, which were very simple: that they were sorry for my loss, that they sent me love. Some people looked terrified when they saw me, as if I might start bleeding on the floor or have some kind of emotional breakdown.

Before I went back to work, a friend warned me that there would definitely be a few people there who wouldn't have found out yet. I was very grateful to the gossip grapevine, to friends and colleagues who spread the word because it was upsetting to get messages from people who didn't know saying, 'I can't wait to see your bump' and 'How's the pregnancy going?'

Counselling helped. I saw a counsellor at my GP's surgery, and a specialist fertility counsellor too. They allowed me to talk about my sadness, guilt and anger. I couldn't let it out at work and I didn't want my husband and friends to think that miscarriage was my only topic of conversation, even though it was very often on my mind.

Q: WHAT DIDN'T HELP?

People saying, 'Don't worry, you can try again.' I know they were well-meaning, but considering the odds of IVF succeeding again, the cost of IVF and that my husband didn't want to try, it upset me. Then there was the acquaintance who said, a few days after the miscarriage, 'My cousin was an older mother too, and her doctor told her that older women like you have to be more careful, take more rest during pregnancy.' I wanted to shout, 'It's a bit fucking late for that.'

Q: IS IT TRUE WHAT PEOPLE SAY, THAT IT GETS EASIER?

In the first weeks after the miscarriage, I couldn't even look at a pregnant woman, pram or pushchair without being convulsed with sadness. Now, two months on, I do still find pregnant women upsetting, but I'm hoping that will go away after my due date comes and goes. And I find only tiny, newborn babies make me sad now, not older ones.

I am still sad at losing that new, little life that was growing inside me. I'd love a baby, and daydream about ways of having one – either by IVF (though we've decided against it, so that's a non-starter), maybe getting pregnant naturally (with no Fallopian tubes, dream on!) or by adoption, although my husband doesn't want to do that.

• • • • • • • • •

Tommy's, the baby charity, run a free telephone helpline for pregnancy loss, as well as maternal health (0800 0147 800) that's staffed by midwives. It's a valuable service, whether you need help on medical or emotional issues.

Your GP may be able to refer you for free counselling; otherwise, find a fertility counsellor at bica.net. I went to see Mollie Graneek, a BICA counsellor who's based in Harley Street and used to be a midwife. The British Association for Counselling & Psychotherapy (BACP.co.uk) has a register of counsellors nationwide; you can search for one near you under categories such as 'bereavement', 'loss' and 'infertility'.

After three miscarriages, your GP should refer you to an NHS specialist for further tests, to find out why you're miscarrying. Some women, especially those who are older, pay to have the tests done privately earlier. Ask your GP or IVF doctor for advice. The Miscarriage Association (miscarriage-association.org.uk) gives advice on investigations and has lots of useful leaflets. You can also leave a message of remembrance for your baby or babies online in their Forget-Me-Not meadow, or sponsor a real tree in Infertility Network UK's Fertility Forest (infertilitynetworkuk.com).

Why I finally stopped IVF

· · · · · · · · · · · ·

What would you pay to have a baby? In the 2010 *Red Annual National Fertility Report*, women said that if IVF were guaranteed to work, they'd be prepared to pay £15,000. In the online world of IVF, you often hear stories of women who've paid that and more, for five, six, eight even 12 cycles. But could you go on that long? Especially as a baby would never be guaranteed?

For me, stopping IVF was harder than discovering that I'd need to have it in the first place. But my husband was adamant that we wouldn't do it again. Logically, I knew he was right, but that didn't stop my grief at losing our last chance of a baby, not least because that chance was taken away from us with a miscarriage. I know that if we didn't have our son, I would have pushed until my husband agreed on a fourth cycle.

So how many cycles do doctors usually suggest? In fact, three cycles is usually considered to be one full treatment. 'You can't expect IVF to work first time,' says Professor Bill

Ledger. 'It's important to realise that IVF isn't just about one cycle, but about three.' The first cycle, he explains, is usually considered a learning curve, where doctors monitor your response to the drugs, and get some idea of the quality of your eggs.

However, if your egg quality is poor or your ovarian reserve is low, your doctor may say that one or two cycles is enough. 'Egg quantity and quality usually go together, so an AMH test or a scan to show your antral follicle count [the number of potential follicles that month] in advance can give you an idea you may get a bad response, and so prevent you putting yourself through the stress and expense of having more treatment that's unlikely to be successful,' says Professor Ledger.

Your chance of getting pregnant on cycles one to three is usually considered to stay the same, according to Mr Tarek El-Toukhy, Consultant and Honorary Lecturer in Reproductive Medicine and Surgery at Guy's and St Thomas' Hospital NHS Foundation Trust. 'But your chances of success are reduced from the fourth cycle onwards,' he says.

'We don't set a limit on the number of cycles in our clinic,' says Professor Ledger. 'We have talked about it, but it seems cruel. If you were on your last go, imagine the stress that would cause. So we leave it to people to make their own minds up. That said, very few do more than three cycles.'

The number of cycles you do may be dictated by your finances. 'That is one of the toughest situations because you don't have a choice,' says Marilyn Crawshaw, retired Senior Lecturer in Social Work and now Honorary Fellow at the University of York. 'It's not unusual for people in this situation to end up at their GP with depression, anxiety or even physical illness as a result,' she says.

You may also make the decision to stop if you are told that your only chance of success is to use technology that doesn't fit with your ethics or religion or with your view of a future family: for example egg or sperm donation.

What's also very hard, says fertility expert Zita West, is when one half of a couple wants to continue, and the other doesn't. 'Couples often clash over how many treatments to have. You may have made a plan at the beginning to do, for example, three treatments,' she says. 'But you can't actually plan until you get there. One partner, usually the woman, may want to keep going, while the other doesn't.'

And because there are always 'miracle' stories about women who conceive after years of trying, it's tempting to keep trying different clinics and treatments. 'Some people go on and on, at the expense of their health, relationships, financial security. And if there is any chance of success, however small, doctors do find it hard to refuse to treat people,' says Zita.

• • • • • • • • •

Gill, 38, is an HR professional from near Huddersfield. She has had two IVF cycles, three donor egg cycles, two miscarriages and an ectopic pregnancy.

Before you've gone through IVF, you think science is fantastic, that it can do anything. But, as my husband Mark and I found out, there aren't always black and white answers when it comes to fertility. At times, that's hard to get your head round.

As a professional, I expect to work for something, and achieve it. But as I discovered, when it comes to your body and to nature, that's not always possible. Not being an expert, in fact sometimes not even knowing the right questions to ask, I found I had to put my full trust in the doctors. That was hard.

We saw our GP after we'd been trying to get pregnant for a year, when I was 34. Initially, we had the usual tests: hormone levels, sperm count and so on, and they all came back fine. Because the doctors thought I might not be ovulating properly, I was put on clomiphene (Clomid), but the scans showed I then produced too many eggs, around four or five each cycle, which meant it was too risky even to try for a pregnancy. That was difficult, to know there were eggs ready, but that we had to do nothing for a month. The doctor tried reducing the dosage, but I kept overstimulating, so he put me on another drug, Tamoxifen. This is usually prescribed to women with breast cancer but, like Clomid, it can stimulate ovulation.

Taking the drugs, I became difficult to live with and very emotional. Mark, to his credit, stayed extremely supportive, even when I was shouting at him in my hormonal ups and downs. He helped as much as he could, coming to appointments with me. And he was there each month when we got the bad news that, yet again, the treatment hadn't worked.

After three unsuccessful cycles of Tamoxifen, the consultant agreed that we could try IVF. We were eligible for two free NHS cycles in our area, but the waiting list was over two years. Given our age, we felt that we couldn't wait that long, so decided to pay.

On the first cycle, I grew eight follicles, and the doctor collected six eggs but, he said, of very poor quality. Even as we were walking to the car park after egg collection, the embryologist called to say they needed to convert from IVF to ICSI because Mark's sperm quality wasn't great either.

I'd joined the support group Infertility Network UK, and logged on that evening to the forum. A few of us having treatment at the same time had become cycle buddies. Even though we were complete strangers, we happily went into personal, physical detail of what we were going through, so we'd formed strong bonds quickly. At times like this, when I was in the depths of despair, my cycle buddies really helped. They would write saying they were feeling the same, or that they had in the past, or even just, 'I understand you'.

Only two embryos survived the night, and we were called in to have a day-two transfer with an hour's notice. It felt like a very negative experience overall, so we weren't very hopeful, although the negative pregnancy test two weeks later was still emotionally crushing.

We had to abandon our second IVF cycle. Just as we were hyped up for egg collection, the final scan showed that, despite being on the highest dose of the stimulation drugs, I'd produced just one follicle. The doctors suggested that we didn't go ahead with collection; the egg was unlikely to survive and, they said, the follicle may not even have had an egg in it. We'd spent £1000 just on the medication on that cycle and, in the end, I had to literally throw away a vial that was worth £200.

I could never quite control my emotions enough to get through treatment unscathed. It was very tough, never knowing what would happen next, how my body would react, if we'd get to the next stage. And then there were the practical considerations, as I tried to minimise my time off work and to keep up a functional, professional image too.

After the second IVF was one of my lowest points. It really did feel as if we'd tried our utmost, gone to the medical profession for help and they'd failed us. In our follow-up consultation, we were told IVF wasn't going to work for us. I was in tears for the whole meeting. All the clinic staff were fantastic and supportive but, in reality, they couldn't make anything better.

Mark was really upset too. In following weeks, we took some proper time out together, walking in the nearby Peak District. We talked through it all, both crying at times. It was hugely helpful in understanding each other and making our next decision. Should we look at egg donation? Or adoption? Or even stop trying altogether?

To help us decide, we had to go back to our dreams of a family and what family meant to us. What we realised was that, for both of us, it was a need to love and nurture children into adulthood. For me, having a family was a reason for being. We were both clear we wanted to keep trying.

For egg donation, we had to come to terms with the fact that only half of the child's genes would come from us. Or there was adoption, where there wouldn't be a biological link to either of us. It didn't seem fair that I didn't have the choice of being biologically related with either option, but I had to accept it, as it was a fact.

We decided on egg donation. I did a lot of research on infertilitynetworkuk.com and another website, fertility-friends.co.uk, and chatted online to women who'd done it. I contacted a number of clinics, both in the UK and abroad, and we made the decision to go to an established clinic with a high success rate in Spain. There, the egg donor has anonymity and she is reimbursed for her time, so there are a lot of younger women doing it and a regular supply of eggs. Unlike the UK at the time, we'd only have to wait a couple of months.

We flew to the clinic for the day. It was lovely: modern and clean, and all the staff were very helpful. That day, we had a consultation, I had a scan and Mark gave a sample.

Back home, there were a lot of forms to fill in and blood tests to organise. It was quite stressful, as it was hard for either of us to make calls during working hours, and there were a few language difficulties, and a delay in replies via email. But the worst aspect of egg donation was the lack of control, part of which was due to Spanish law being so strict about donor anonymity. You are told when your donor starts stimulating, so you can inject down-regulating drugs to match your cycle to hers. You're also given an indication of the date you'll fly out for egg collection, if all goes well. But you're only told that date for certain a maximum of 48 hours before.

Our first cycle was abandoned because the donor didn't produce enough eggs. More tears and frustration. We then had to wait a couple of months for my body to recover after the down-regulation and to be matched with a different donor.

Finally, we started our second cycle with a new donor. The day before egg collection, we were told that we needed to be in Spain at 7 p.m. the following day for Mark's sperm to fertilise the donor's eggs. While the egg collection produced nine eggs, we soon had another letdown: by the time the embryos could be transferred into me, there were just two left.

But, unbelievably, two weeks later, we had a positive pregnancy test. Although it didn't feel like a proper pregnancy because my beta hCG levels were on the low side, and weren't rising as they should. A couple of weeks later, I miscarried over Christmas. Even though I'd felt something wasn't right all along, it was upsetting all the same, an awful Christmas.

That New Year, we had a few bottles of wine to commiserate, and I cried a lot. I was able to book counselling through work, so I had four sessions on my own and two with Mark. The counsellor was fantastic, really helping me to deal with some of the anger I had against myself and my body, to get over the waste of money and to come to terms with the grief.

We decided to continue with egg-donation treatment, but in the UK this time. We found out that the waiting list for donor egg IVF in a clinic a couple of hours' drive from us was only a few months. Most of their donor eggs came from egg sharing, where the sharer gets free IVF in return for donating half her eggs.

The first cycle was pretty awful. The sharer produced 10 eggs but only four were mature enough to fertilise, so each couple got just two. This is quite unusual so, yet again, it felt as if luck was against us.

The day after egg collection, the clinic rang us to ask us to come in early for the transfer: as there were only two embryos, they felt they would be better off in my uterus than in a petri dish. It was hugely disappointing and I spent a lot of the drive up to have the transfer crying. Because the embryos were put in early, we had no idea of their grade or quality. I did get pregnant, but again, my hCG levels weren't quite right as they went up too slowly. We were due to go camping in Cornwall but, after looking at the numbers, the consultant told us there was a chance this pregnancy was ectopic, so it was too dangerous for me to go.

For two weeks, it was still too early to see whether the pregnancy was in my womb or my Fallopian tubes. Finally, a doctor found the pregnancy in my right tube. I had surgery to remove it along with my Fallopian tube later that day. It felt as though for each of the cycles we'd had, something different had gone wrong. We'd had abandoned cycles, miscarriage cycles and now an ectopic pregnancy.

On our very last cycle, also egg-donor IVF, the miscarriage happened just before my seven-week scan, at Christmas again. That was the most devastating of all because, until then, my hCG levels were more than doubling every 48 hours, as they're supposed to. In fact, they were so good that we'd actually dared to think it might be twins.

Before that last cycle, my way of dealing with IVF not working had been to keep looking forward and to be hopeful.

But this time, I felt different. At the beginning, you never imagine having to give up, but something had changed inside me. I knew the time had come to stop treatment, but I wasn't clear on what to do next. I went for counselling again (arranged through my GP) to help me move on. I did feel some relief, but it was also scary because treatment had been part of my life for so long.

By making the decision to go through egg donation, I'd accepted our child wouldn't be biologically related to me, so moving on from there to adoption was quite quick for me. It took Mark a little longer. But, after a lot of talking, we agreed that while we'd never be biological parents, we'd still be great, loving, supportive parents to children who need that love.

Eighteen months on, we've been approved for adoption and, in a few weeks, we'll go to matching panel, hopefully to adopt two children – siblings – if things go smoothly. I'm enjoying the feeling that we're moving forward, and am very hopeful that we will have our family one day soon.

We were both slightly nervous about adoption at first, not about our decision, but about the unknown. What issues might a child or children have? Would we be able to cope? What age would be right for us? But we've worked through all that with the help of pre-adoption training and the home study. What we've been through, and how it made us talk to each other, has helped a lot in making those big decisions.

Sadly for us, we are part of the group who come away from fertility treatment empty of pocket and with empty arms. We tried harder than most people, but it didn't happen. Out of the friends I met online at the IN UK website, I'm the only one who hasn't had a baby. At times, it makes me sad that it had to be me, but I can't do anything about it.

Trying for babies and IVF was a huge part of my life for so long. I lost my 30s to it. I do feel a bit jealous of women having IVF now, as I don't have that option any more. And, in fact, recent blood tests showed I have a condition – I'm lupus anticoagulant positive – which could explain the miscarriages. That has finally stopped any further thoughts of IVF.

Given our time again, I'd start treatment much earlier. Apart from that, there is very little I would change – except the outcome. We made some fantastic friends through IVF and we also found out how great some of our non-IVF friends are. Although I would never wish what we've been through on anyone else, looking back, I can see it brought Mark and I closer together. There's some truth in the saying, 'what doesn't kill you, makes you stronger'.

Q: HOW DID YOU KNOW WHEN TO STOP TREATMENT?

At the age of 37, after six cycles of Clomid, five IVF cycles, three failed pregnancies in a year, and having spent over £20,000, I knew it was over. I never, ever thought I'd give up, but after the fight and determination I'd showed over three years of trying, this time felt different. We knew we couldn't keep putting ourselves through more financial pressure, more waiting lists, more drugs, more uncertainty. I felt defeated, and knew the time had come. It was a gut feeling. I didn't know before the fifth cycle, but I knew very quickly afterwards. It took slightly longer for Mark, I think because I was so emotionally and physically affected by the miscarriages.

Q: WHAT'S YOUR ADVICE TO ANYONE CONSIDERING EGG DONATION IN SPAIN?

It's to be certain you're happy with the legal situation on the anonymity of the donor there. Our clinic took it extremely seriously and shared very little information with us. That means you only get 48 hours' notice of when you need to fly out, which was fine when the cycle went smoothly. But when the first Spanish cycle was abandoned because the donor didn't stimulate enough, we waited 10 days after we'd expected to travel before they emailed to tell us. I'm a very organised, well-planned person, so that was hard.

Q: HOW DID COUNSELLING HELP AFTER YOU REACHED YOUR DECISION?

It was what got me through. I did a lot of crying, used a lot of tissues. I was angry that I'd had to go through infertility, and also at the money we'd wasted. I was angry at my body too, as I felt as if it had turned on me.

When we got married, we didn't think we'd have to go through the indignities of IVF. It's made us a very strong couple, especially as we've made sure we've kept talking. With the help of counselling, support from friends and family and my husband, I've been able to bring myself out of my unhappiness. Counselling helped me to see that some people would have crumbled in my position, but I realised that I should feel proud that I fought so long and hard for a family. The loss of our pregnancies will always be with us, but we can cope with that now. It's become a part of who we are.

• • • • • • • • •

When you look at whether it's worth continuing with more cycles of IVF, it depends which study you look at. One, from the US, which looked at 300,000 cycles, showed that the likelihood of getting pregnant dropped after two cycles (although there was still a chance). Another, from Australia, stated that for maximum chance of pregnancy, it's worth having five cycles.

If only there was a quiz you could take with questions on your emotions, finances and likelihood of getting pregnant. And, once you filled it in, it could tell you whether it's time to stop treatment. Or whether you should carry on and try egg or sperm donation or surrogacy. Or start the adoption process or fostering. Or decide to live child-free. But life is more complicated than that, of course. Counselling can help you make a decision (find a specialist infertility counsellor at bica.net).

There's a really honest and moving account of one couple's decision to stop having treatment on one of the *New York Times* parenting blogs (see http://parenting.blogs.nytimes.com/2009/09/10/life-after-infertility-treatments-fail/). Shelagh Little says: 'Every woman facing infertility has to decide when she's had enough, when she has reached her ethical, emotional and/or financial edge ... I needed to stop trying so I could get back to living.'

There's more advice from blogger Laurie Pawlik-Kienlen at http://theadventurouswriter.com/blogbaby/should-i-stop-trying-to-get-pregnant-ending-infertility-treatments/ (theadventurouswriter.com/blogbaby has all kinds of articles on fertility). She outlines reasons for stopping, including emotional exhaustion, not being able to afford treatment, feeling as if you've wasted years of your life on fertility, and the fact that other aspects of your life are suffering.

I moved on to
a child-free life

● ● ● ● ● ● ● ● ● ● ● ●

T he patient group Infertility Network UK estimate that
half of those who have IVF stop having treatment
without having had a baby, although some do go on
to get pregnant naturally. Stopping can bring feelings of
relief, but also of loss, sadness and grief that can be extremely
painful and run very deep.

The trouble is, it's not often a decision you actually make,
but can be forced on you because you've run out of money or
your partner wants to stop. 'I've known people who have felt
as if life isn't worth living when they feel the decision was
made for them,' says Marilyn Crawshaw, fertility counsellor
and Honorary Fellow in Social Work at the University
of York.

If you think that your next cycle will be your last or you've
finally stepped off the treatment conveyor belt, what can
help? Counselling, for one. 'Some people in this situation can
feel "stuck",' says Crawshaw. 'They don't want to let go of
their wish to become parents, but can't yet move towards

building an alternative life, as that too feels unbearable. During counselling, I can tell them about others I've worked with in their position who eventually were able to move on to a fulfilling life. They may not be able to believe it for themselves at that point, but I think it can help to know that others have managed it.'

Sheena Young of Infertility Network UK, who herself came out of fertility treatment without a baby, now works with IN UK's support group for those in the same situation, More To Life. She says that if you don't want to use counselling to manage your experience, contact with others in the same situation – such as the get-togethers organised by More To Life – can be life-changing. 'Just to be able to say to other people, for example, "My sister is pregnant again and I don't know how to handle it", and for them to understand how you feel, is valuable.'

The key to being able to move on, according to Sheena, often has a lot to do with how and why you stopped having treatment. 'The satisfactory ending of treatment isn't just about whether you have a baby,' she says. It may be easier to move on if, for example, your doctor has made a firm clinical judgment that it's time to stop. 'Sometimes clinicians are not always as helpful as they could be at saying "stop", and telling you that if IVF was going to work it would have worked by now,' says Sheena. 'Being told that, you may be angry, but it also forces you into thinking what to do next.'

No one plans to have 10 treatments when they start out, but it's difficult to move on when there's even a tiny bit of hope. 'When I was having IVF, we'd decide to stop, then we'd learn about a new treatment that might work,' says Sheena, 'then away we'd go again. And the more times we did this, the harder it was to stop in the end.'

The adjustment to a new life, a new image of yourself is – inevitably – not a quick process. 'The first year, you're probably only getting over the fact the treatment has ended,' says Sheena. 'You have to learn to live with the disappointment. My husband and I always tried to stay positive, and focused on what we did have – a good marriage. It takes a long time; not to fill the gap left by children, but to fill your life in a way that makes you feel fulfilled.'

· · · · · · · · ·

Jane, 36, is a music teacher from Derbyshire. Her husband Andrew had had a vasectomy before they met.

Lying on a yoga mat under dimmed lights, eyes closed, head on a pillow and covered with a fluffy brown blanket, I breathed slowly – in for a count of four, and out for a count of four. Along with six other women who were trying to conceive, I was at a fertility meditation and visualisation class.

The teacher had a lovely voice, really calm and restful, as she told me to think of myself walking through a wood, imagining all the sensations I'd be feeling and what I'd be seeing. Then she moved on to helping me visualise opening my body to becoming pregnant.

After the failure of our third IVF cycle, I'd started trying different ways I thought might make my body more receptive to pregnancy. Whether relaxation and positive thinking actually makes any difference or not I don't know, but it made me feel better (as did my weekly acupuncture sessions). Some weeks at the class, I might feel quite emotional and teary. Most of the time, I felt positive and came out feeling very relaxed.

It had taken me weeks to get over every treatment failure. Andrew had been upset too, and I know he found it hard that he couldn't do anything to make me feel better. And I suppose because he'd been married before, and his vasectomy was the original reason we had to have ICSI, he felt responsible in some way. Even when later tests showed that I had issues too, he wanted to blame himself.

The first ICSI cycle seemed to go well: eggs which fertilised correctly, good-quality embryos to put back in. But the result was a negative pregnancy test. The consultant we saw afterwards could find no particular reason why it didn't work, so we decided to try again. Andrew was less keen than me: he didn't like seeing me so upset after the failure.

The next cycle, I was even more anxious because we'd already paid out £3000 for the first treatment with nothing to show for it. That's a lot of money to spend getting nowhere. I was also nervous of what I was doing to my body by taking so many drugs.

My physical response to the second cycle was pretty much the same as the first cycle – a decent number of good eggs and embryos. But the two-week wait was even more nerve-wracking this time. I found there was an argument going on, constantly, in my head. One voice was saying, I really want to have a family, I want this to work so much and I can't think of anything more amazing than being pregnant. But the other one was saying, I'm not a hundred per cent convinced this is *ever* going to work with me. I tried to block out my negative thoughts as much as possible, but when I was on my own, or when I went to bed, they came back. The second treatment ended in another negative pregancy test.

For our third cycle, we decided to try the embryos that had been frozen from the first cycle. That cycle was much easier: fewer scans, less prodding and poking and not nearly as many drugs. This time, a blood test showed I was pregnant. But when the nurse called to tell us, she warned me that my levels of pregnancy hormone – beta hCG – weren't very high, although all I heard was the word 'positive', and got overexcited. We thought everything was going to be fine, so we told friends and family our news, and everyone else then got excited for us too. But the next blood test, a couple of days later, showed the hCG levels weren't going up as expected. Finally, 10 days later, we had a scan, which showed there was nothing in my womb.

We went away for the weekend to the Lake District, just to be somewhere different. Then, the next day, I had a call from the clinic to say that my hCG levels weren't dropping as they should have been with a miscarriage, and there was a possibility it was an ectopic pregnancy. The clinic said that I needed to be monitored closely, as an ectopic can be dangerous if the growing embryo ruptures the Fallopian tube. So we drove home quickly, and went straight to our local A&E. We arrived there at 8 p.m. on Saturday evening, and they kept me in overnight.

The following day, scans still didn't show anything – it was too early. I was discharged, but had to go back for more hCG blood tests. A few days later, doctors decided that it was an ectopic pregnancy, and I had an injection of methotrexate, which kills any embryonic cells. My mum and Andrew came with me, and they were hugely supportive, but I couldn't help feeling like I was the only who'd ever gone through this, and no one else could understand.

I still had to go back for hCG blood tests every few days, to make sure my levels were going down. That was horrible, as the tests were done at the pregnancy clinic, so I was often surrounded in the waiting room by obviously pregnant women. I did a lot of crying in the car park.

It took me a few months to feel calmer emotionally. But the promise of having got a positive test was a temptation to keep going. We called our clinic and they said there were further tests we could have. They specialise in a controversial area of fertility called reproductive immunology. It looks at how your immune system is functioning and whether it's to blame for your embryos not implanting.

Andrew's tests all came back fine, but I had few slightly abnormal results. The consultant at the clinic suggested that on our next cycle, I should take some more drugs for this: steroids, low-dose aspirin and a blood-thinning drug Clexane (enoxaparin), and possibly have a treatment called intravenous immunoglobulin (IVIg).

It seemed like every time we had a barrier, the clinic would tell us that they could fix it. Probably, we just weren't listening when they told us the negatives. The extra drugs were a sticking point between Andrew and me, as he thought I was putting enough into my body already, but a year later, we felt ready to start another cycle. By this time, my brother had had his first baby and was expecting another one, and a lot of friends were starting their families too. I tried to be a good auntie and friend, but it was becoming harder for me.

Andrew and I decided I'd take the steroids, but not have the IVIg, because it's a blood product and that concerned us. It's also extremely expensive. That's when I started having acupuncture and doing the visualisation classes. The treatment went really well, and we got excellent embryos, like before. When I had them put back in, I did my visualisation exercises religiously. I felt I'd done everything to give this IVF the maximum chance of working. All through the two-week wait, I really thought I might be pregnant.

The day before we were due to have a blood test at the clinic, I did a home test and it was positive. I felt like the happiest person in the world when I showed Andrew. We didn't stop smiling the whole day. We went to the clinic and the hCG blood test showed a really high positive too.

But then, a week later, I started spotting. The clinic told me all I could do was to rest, and to wait until I could have a scan. At six weeks, a scan showed a sac and a foetal pole, which is the very earliest sign of a baby. There was no heartbeat, but the consultant said it was still early on, so we should wait.

At a scan a week later, there was even less to see, and definitely no heartbeat. In one second, we went from being on top of the world to as low as we could get. Leaving the clinic, I could barely walk. I had to sit down, I was sobbing so hard. It felt unbelievably unfair, cruel and painful. The whole thing had been so nerve-wracking and draining; the expectation of being pregnant each time, and telling people, and getting so excited, then the let-down.

Andrew and I had to tell everyone, again, that the pregnancy had gone wrong. In a sense, it did help to get messages saying, 'I'm so sorry, I hope you're ok', but having to describe what had happened was awful.

I really had felt as if all I'd done would pay off this time. I felt as if we deserved it, that we'd been through enough. The clinic told me I should just let nature take its course, and my body would expel the pregnancy naturally, but it didn't happen. Waiting felt like an eternity. After 10 days I went, in floods of tears, to my GP who called the hospital and booked me in for an ERPC (evacuation of retained products of conception), and I had the pregnancy removed under general anaesthetic.

We decided to take some time out from treatment. I was struggling, crying a lot. I wanted to be by myself and I shut everybody out, even Andrew. I didn't want to be the person who talked about IVF all the time, so I didn't talk about it at all. That meant people probably thought I was coping, so they didn't ask. With hindsight, I should have talked to friends and family more. I expected too much of everybody – that they'd understand completely; I can see now that I wasn't being realistic.

I felt like nobody understood how I felt, completely empty and alone, and guilty that we'd failed. I'd go through stages of feeling angry that we'd almost got there, but it had been taken away, and upset with myself, then I'd wonder what had I done wrong and blame myself. Then I'd feel upset and that it was unfair, as everyone else we knew who was having treatment had managed to come out the other side. I remember having a stupid thought that if a friend who had twins could have had just one, I could have had one, and that would have been fair. I went through a whole self-loathing stage, where I hated what I was and what I looked like, and my sex drive disappeared too.

I went back to see my GP, who told me I was on the edge of being depressed, and signed me off work for a few weeks. She offered me antidepressants, but I didn't want to take them. I was going to the clinic for counselling, where the counsellor's approach was to listen and be a sounding board, which suited me at the time as I had a lot to get out of my system, mostly anger. Poor Andrew ended up as a bit of a punch bag. But I knew he wouldn't leave me. He just put up with it – bless him. I was horrible over the smallest things, even what we were having for dinner. Although it was awful for everyone around me, I needed to go through this grieving process.

It was probably four months before I began to feel more like myself; the worst four months of my life. I've never had such sadness and anger, before or since. Andrew booked a holiday to Scotland, to a beautiful part of the Highlands where we did a lot of walking and talking. In such a peaceful place, I started to feel a bit more human, a bit more happy and a bit more like myself.

It may sound stupid, but I still didn't feel as if I'd spent long enough being sad; it was such a big deal. There's no rule book that says: you must be sad for X number of weeks after a miscarriage.

It wasn't until a month after our holiday that we actually addressed the issue of having another try. We had two frozen embryos left over from the fourth cycle – both good quality. I felt that our embryos were just waiting to see if we were going to use them. After everything, I was expecting to have to fight my corner with Andrew to have treatment, but he already seemed to know that I was determined.

So we went for one last try. But on the day the embryos were thawed, the clinic called to say that neither of them had made it. I wasn't expecting that. It was a complete anti-climax; all of a sudden, we were left with nothing. It didn't feel right to finish like that.

I went back for two more counselling sessions at the clinic, but I began to hate going there. It didn't feel right, going to the place where I'd had treatment to talk about the fact that I was stopping.

My GP put me in touch with a therapist who specialises in cognitive behavioural therapy (CBT). Her advice was very useful. She taught me how to get out the cycle of feeling bad and blaming myself for failure, when what had happened was, in fact, out of my control. She showed me how to deal with difficult situations, to train myself into positive thinking. And she made me see that my thoughts were separate from what was actually happening. That was a revelation to me. CBT lifted my mood and my confidence.

We did a lot of work on communication and being assertive. I was having problems talking to Andrew about my feelings. Not talking was making us feel further apart, which in turn made me sad and feel worse about our relationship. With the therapist, I worked on how to talk without becoming confrontational or negative. That helped put our relationship back together again.

One of the main things I struggled with was my self-image now I wasn't going to be a mum, and what would give me meaning in life. I learned that in the past, I'd given parenthood a huge emphasis, but that when I put being a mum in context with everything else that I did and had, it was just one part of me. Parenthood didn't have to overshadow everything else.

Now, 18 months later, the difficult moments are much l ess frequent. Having talked to other people who've been through the same thing but who are 10 or 20 years ahead of me. I've accepted that there will always be some sadness, but it becomes part of who you are instead of defining you.

It's really easy to come out of IVF feeling as if you're the only one who has failed. So I joined a support group called More To Life, for people who don't end up becoming parents. I started by going on the online forums then graduated to local get-togethers, lunch or tea or a weekend away. Eighteen months later, I'm now the county organiser.

Recently, I met up with a new member, and we talked about her IVF. I came away thinking that not being a mum can still hurt sometimes, but also realising how far I've come. It's amazing that I managed to survive such a difficult time, and can now be strong for other people too.

There are four very special children in my life: my three nieces and my nephew. I see them regularly and really enjoy the relationships I have with them. We saw my sister and her daughters, aged one and three, yesterday. They're gorgeous, but really full-on. Afterwards, I said to Andrew, 'I'm really glad we don't have to cope with that amount of noise and madness every day.'

I am grateful for what I've got now because I've almost got the best of both worlds; the company of children when I want, but our quiet, peaceful house and our dog when I don't.

I feel quite contented. It would have been lovely to have a family, but we have a really good life.

Q: WHAT HELPED YOU AT THE END OF YOUR INFERTILITY JOURNEY?

After we decided to stop treatment, I joined a support group called More To Life. From meeting people in the online forums, I learned that people feel bad after giving up IVF for different reasons – maybe not carrying on the family line, maybe not fulfilling a desire to be a mother. It's a powerful thing to have contact with other people in the same situation, not having to explain yourself or feeling like you don't belong. At our get-togethers, we don't necessarily talk about the fact that we're childless – we've got plenty of other common ground – but it is comfortable not having to talk about children or listen to people talk about theirs.

Q: SHOULD YOU HAVE STOPPED EARLIER?

I've known women who've gone through five, seven and nine cycles. At the beginning, I thought, I could never do that. And then all of a sudden I was on number four, and it turned out it wasn't so hard to get to that stage, after all. I do think that if I'd stopped after our third treatment, when we first talked about it, I would've felt cheated.

Q: HOW DID YOU KNOW IT WAS TIME TO STOP TREATMENT?

I felt as if I'd put my body through enough pain and I'd put myself through enough heartbreak and disappointment. And we were running out of money. Adding everything up, we'd spent at least £10,000, maybe more. It didn't feel right to keep going. Much as it was tempting to think, 'I'll just have another try', I knew it wasn't that easy.

Q: WHAT WAS THE MOST USEFUL COGNITIVE BEHAVIOURAL THERAPY TECHNIQUE YOU USED?

Keeping a thought diary. In the first column, I had to write down what I was thinking and feeling. In the second, I wrote what it was about the situation that made me feel bad. Then, in the third, I had to separate what was real, and what were simply my thoughts. Eventually, I learned to do that without writing it down.

So, for example, once I got angry when I heard a pregnant woman moaning about her back hurting and not getting any sleep, and how she couldn't wait not to be pregnant. After doing the thought diary, I realised that she wasn't trying to hurt me personally, and I was being oversensitive.

• • • • • • • • •

The UK's leading organisation for those who are unintentionally childless is More To Life (infertilitynetworkuk/more-tolife). For a small fee, you get access to a professional telephone advice line and other support via chat rooms, and regional meet-ups. 'How wonderful it was to go to a social event and not be asked whether you have kids,' says Julie, a member. They also have factsheets, including 'Moving on to a Positive Life Without Children', which stresses that you need to get to know yourself again after spending all your time and energy on trying to get pregnant. And from the US, Pamela Tsigdinos blogs on all aspects of childlessness, including talking to friends and family and stopping treatment at www.coming2terms.com. She's also author of the award-winning book *Silent Sorority* (BookSurge Publishing). Other recommended books are: *Pink for a Girl* (Hay House), Isla McGuckin's personal experience of unexplained fertility and *Beyond Childlessness* by Rachel Black and Louise Scull (Rodale).

If you'd like to commemorate a failed cycle or miscarriage, you could dedicate a tree in Infertility Network UK's Fertility Forest, in conjunction with the Woodland Trust. 'Turn the experience of infertility into something positive, and help the environment at the same time,' says IN UK (see the fertility forest button on the homepage of infertilitynetworkuk.com).

Why I adopted
after IVF

. . . .

How can you know if adoption might be the way to create your family? 'My advice is to try to work out how much *parenthood* itself matters to you, rather than *biological* parenthood,' says Marilyn Crawshaw, co-editor of *Adopting After Infertility*. She says around three-quarters of people who turn to adoption do so because of infertility. 'But if you instinctively know that parenthood is what matters to you, that is what will take you towards adoption.'

When you first start looking into adoption, you may still be thinking of it as second best. 'If you adopt, you've had to put aside your first choice, which was to have some biological connection in the family,' says Crawshaw. Maya, whose story is below, confesses that it wasn't until partway through the adoption process that she accepted she wasn't going to have a child who was related to her.

Then there's the fact that you have to accept not being pregnant, not knowing your child as a newborn or even as a baby or toddler, depending on the age of the child you adopt. Social workers also routinely warn that any child who's been in care may be damaged in some way. Or you may be put off by the stories in the media of adoption gone wrong or scare stories of red tape and bad practices.

Finally, even once you've decided to go ahead, the adoption process itself can feel very intrusive into your personal life, and it can take months or even a year or two from beginning to end. 'Adoption really does have to move to being your first choice, as it's extremely difficult to go through the process unless you are really committed to it,' says Crawshaw. 'What you have to realise is that adoption agencies are there to meet the children's needs, not yours – and that's how it should be after all,' says Crawshaw. 'Then you can make sense of the preparation process. And, if you get approved, the good news is that your chance of becoming parents is extremely high, as the agencies don't invest time and money into people unless they're going to use them. And that's when the really good part starts – the vast majority of adoptive parents find parenthood every bit as rewarding as any other parent.'

• • • • • • • • •

Maya, 41, a property manager from London, wanted to continue with IVF but her husband Tom, 47, thought it was time to stop.

Lying on a sunbed on the white sand of one of the most beautiful beaches in Mauritius, looking at the turquoise sea, I felt relaxed for the first time in ages. Tom and I finally had the time and space to talk about the fact that, a month before, our second IVF cycle had ended in failure.

'I don't want us to go through IVF again,' Tom said. He told me that he'd found it very hard to be around me when I was having fertility treatment – that it had made me nervous and uncharacteristically irritable. And that he'd found every one of our six failed IUI cycles and two IVF cycles very hard emotionally too. And, he said, he couldn't bear to see me going through hell every time the treatments didn't work.

That Tom was completely certain that he wanted to stop was a surprise to me. And I was even more shocked when he told me that he had felt like that for a while. At our follow-up consultation, our IVF doctor had told us that, in his opinion, there wasn't a good reason for us to continue with treatment. He said I wasn't producing enough eggs to make it a worthwhile option. Unless we wanted to use donor eggs, he explained, we had an extremely low chance of pregnancy.

My first thought was, 'He has no right to tell us to stop.' I was devastated. I'm a very calm person normally but, walking out of his office, I was furious as well as upset. I wanted to find another clinic that would treat us straight away. Because we'd had an ectopic pregnancy from our first cycle of IVF, I kept thinking it was possible for me to get pregnant, that it was worth us carrying on.

For me, donor eggs were an immediate no-no, and I said so in the consultation. Instinctively, the thought of someone else's eggs being put together with Tom's sperm felt wrong. I was still focused on doing IVF with my eggs. I knew the consultant's opinion meant a lot to Tom, that he trusted him, but on the way home from the hospital in the car, I told Tom we should try again, that we still had a chance. I said that I didn't mind going through IVF again if, at the end, we had a baby. Logically, I knew the doctor was being reasonable, but I didn't want to hear it.

I knew that Tom had always been keen on adoption; he'd brought it up as a serious possibility even while we were doing IUI. He had close friends who had adopted, so he'd seen it could have a happy ending. To go along with him at the time, but hoping that it would never come to that, I'd agreed adoption was a good idea. But when Tom brought up adoption for a second time, on the beach, I was still determined to carry on trying for our own biological baby. It was only when he said he felt that IVF had been undermining our relationship that I started to reconsider. I knew that more IVF would put pressure on our financial situation too and, deep down, I knew the consultant was right.

Our relationship was more important to me than anything, so I listened to what Tom said. To be honest, I think I needed him to be so definite so that I could move on myself. He did also say that if I really wanted to carry on with IVF, he would support me, so he didn't force me into making a decision. But, as we talked, I realised that adopting would be better for us and our relationship, and agreed to start the process. I have to confess that I was still struggling inside and, in my mind, a tiny hope remained that I might get pregnant naturally.

We are a mixed-race couple so, a few months later, we went to an open evening run by an adoption agency which specialises in black, Asian and mixed-race children. That was when adoption began to seem real. I realised that in my desire for a baby I'd been thinking only of myself but in fact, we might be able to give a home to a child who needed one.

The next step was a three-day preparation group, which we attended with other couples. That's when we found out more about the possible issues that children in care can face. I discovered that a child aged just two might have been moved from one foster placement to another six or seven times and was likely to have suffered neglect or abuse. I found that sad and scary.

Even though I knew that any child we adopted would not have had a great start in life, somehow that didn't put me off.

In fact, the more I found out about how and why children get taken into care, the stronger and more able to cope I felt.

The next step was the assessment process. A social worker came to our home every week for two months, asking us very personal questions. We had to share every detail about the kind of upbringing we'd had and important times in our lives and describe our parenting values, our support network and how we lived as a couple.

To start with, it felt very invasive. But through the process I got to know myself better and I learned things about Tom. I told the social worker that when I was five, and my sister came along, I felt resentful. I was surprised to see that appear in the social worker's final report with quite a lot of emphasis, as I'd thought it was normal childish behaviour. But, generally, as neither of us had anything to hide, we were happy to be open.

We then had to fill out more forms, get CRB (Criminal Record Bureau) checked, have medicals, nominate friends to be interviewed about our suitability as parents and, finally, go in front of a panel of a dozen 'worthies', a group whose job it was to play God. They would decide whether we were fit to parent – or not. Twenty minutes after being asked a few relatively easy questions by them, our nervous feelings were replaced by one of pure joy. We had been passed by the panel and were now officially 'prospective adoptive parents'.

Just a week later, we were put on a shortlist of three families to adopt a child, a two-year-old girl. We saw a photo and were told some basic information: her name and where she lived. We thought there was a good chance she'd be placed with us but, after a lot of toing and froing, we got another call: she wasn't going to any of the three, after all. The report said the decision was made because my side of the family didn't live in the UK, we didn't have a garden and we didn't have the experience to look after a two-year-old.

We couldn't understand it; all that information was already in our report, even before we'd been put on the shortlist. And the thought of that little girl staying in care was even harder to accept than the IVF failures. Tom and I made a big fuss, writing letters to the social workers. After a while, we realised it was stupid to keep torturing ourselves about her – she wasn't going to be our little girl, no matter how much we wanted her. After a few months, we found out she had been placed with another couple and that allowed us to move on.

Then, the social workers got back in touch with details of another little girl from a different local authority – Aurelie, who was also two. They sent a video of her. Tom fell in love straight away, but I wasn't so sure. I said that I didn't like the way she was dressed, but it's more likely, I think, that I was scared, just in case we weren't judged suitable to be her parents. It took a couple of weeks for me to allow myself to know she was right for us.

The matching panel, which was held in an institutional meeting room, was comprised of a dozen people who would decide if this little girl would become our daughter. It was extremely daunting but, as we had all the way through, we tried to be ourselves when we answered their questions. While they made their decision, we went into a meeting room next door to wait. We held hands, too nervous to speak much. When they called us back in to say we were matched, I couldn't stop crying, I was so happy. I kept saying that it was a miracle.

Before we could meet Aurelie, we made a book of photos for her foster carers to show her, introducing ourselves and our family and explaining that we were her new mummy and daddy. We also made her a video of a teddy showing her round what would be her new house, especially her bedroom, which we'd decorated, her new little bed and all her new toys.

Just two weeks after being 'approved', we went to meet Aurelie for the first time. She was sitting on her foster carer's lap in the garden, waiting for us. She was very cute and extremely shy, but she mumbled, 'Are you my new mummy and daddy?' We melted.

We gave her the teddy wrapped up, and even as she opened it, she knew it was the one she'd seen in the video and she took 'Nounours' for a walk around the garden. We stayed more than an hour that first day, and even then I didn't want to leave. She had been with the same foster carers for most of her life, and they obviously loved her very much, so our first impression was of a happy little girl.

Over the next week, we got to know Aurelie. Each visit, we built up our time with her slowly. We started taking her to a nearby park, and she went on a slide for the first time, which she adored. The second week, she came to our house with her foster carers. Once she'd settled in, they left her with us for the day. When she saw her bedroom, she knew this was her new home, the one she'd seen in the video. She lay on the bed, happily cuddling the toy animals.

Three days later, we picked her up for the last time. After a quick 10-minute goodbye to her foster carers, she was in the car and our lives had suddenly changed. I didn't have time to worry about how it was going. We were thrust into the roles of being parents to a bright and inquisitive two-year-old.

With her foster carers, Aurelie hadn't gone to bed before 10 p.m., but we started a routine of 6 p.m. tea, then bath, bed, story and sleep. The first night, she woke up screaming at 2 a.m. That was our first real 'Help!' moment. We sat by her bed and she looked at us, obviously thinking: what on earth is happening? We held her close, then I lay next to her and I pretended to go to sleep. After five minutes I could hear her gently snoring beside me.

Every evening, we would stick to the same routine, and she soon got used to it. Meanwhile, we got used to her too. We bonded very quickly and now, 10 months on, she's so relaxed that she can even afford to be naughty! She's going to nursery three days a week now, and loves it as there's so much to do there.

Aurelie is now very much part of our wider family too – my mother, who often comes to stay, and Tom's parents, his brothers and sister, not to mention their children, all love the new addition. And the incredible news is that our family is going to get bigger; a few weeks ago, we were told that we are going to be able to adopt her baby half brother, so our family will be complete. In fact, I said to Tom the other day that we'll need to be careful with contraception, as if I got pregnant now it would stop us adopting our little boy!

We are so settled and happy that I can admit to myself now I was never sure that adoption would work. You do hear some bad stories, and you wonder if that's going to happen. But, so far, we feel we are the luckiest parents in the world, and that we are blessed in ways we couldn't have imagined.

Q: DO YOU REGRET THAT YOU WEREN'T ABLE TO CARRY YOUR CHILDREN?

When we were trying, I used to dread the subject of babies coming up when we were at family events. Around the time I was trying to conceive, it seemed as if everyone in Tom's family was giving birth. Even when we were first looking into adoption, I found it really hard to be around pregnant women because it reminded me that I'd never know what it felt like to be pregnant. Since Aurelie arrived, I don't feel like that at all.

Q: HOW DID YOU KNOW WHEN TO STOP HAVING TREATMENT?

Even though I didn't want to stop after our second IVF, I had to listen to Tom. I was desperate. I loved children so much, which made it very hard not to have one. I was clinging to a tiny hope that the next cycle, I'd get pregnant naturally. Tom listened when the doctor said that I didn't produce enough eggs, and it wasn't worth us carrying on with IVF. Eventually, I had to accept that he was right.

Q: WOULD YOU RECOMMEND ADOPTION?

It isn't easy. It's a journey with lots of twists and turns, but I'd do it again, without doubt. I've met a lot of other adoptive parents who feel the same way. They inspired us to carry on when things seemed hopeless, and now we have been rewarded with our own special family. And although the assessment process is intrusive and it does take a long time, I'd still recommend adoption wholeheartedly. It's the best thing I have ever done. There are so many children out there who need a home, and one of them might be yours.

· · · · · · · · ·

Maya says she found the British Agencies for Fostering and Adoption website very useful (BAAF: baaf.org.uk and 020 7421 2671). There are lots of stories on their blog, too, at baafadoption.blogspot.com. Their offshoot website, bemyparent.org.uk has biogs of children who need families (if they don't make you want to adopt, nothing will!), as well as a quiz that answers lots of common questions on adoption.

IN UK have two adoption factsheets: one on adoption in the UK, and one from abroad; both are very comprehensive about the process and red tape of adoption, as well as the emotional issues. And information from the government is available at direct.gov.uk/en/Parents/AdoptionAndFostering/index.htm.

Dr Marilyn Crawshaw has co-edited a book that covers multiple aspects of adoption, called *Adopting After Infertility* (Jessica Kingsley Publishers). Although it's an academic book, it gives a useful overview of adoption, and would help a potential adoptive parent to understand the actual process from the point of view of the professionals working in adoption too.

Afterword

● ● ● ● ● ● ● ● ● ● ●

O ne day, when you've finished having fertility treatment, and, hopefully, have the family you want, you'll look back at this time of your life and think: I made it.

When I first started interviewing the 22 women in this book, I was in quite a bad place after a biochemical pregnancy. But interviewing them, hearing their most personal feelings and memories, got me back on the right track and allowed me to steel myself for a last IVF treatment.

The intention of writing this book is that it will do the same for you: get you through any hard times, help you to know what to expect, and where to get the advice and support you need too.

During my treatments, I was fortunate enough to have support from some of the UK's leading experts. I am particularly indebted to fertility expert Zita West and specialist fertility acupuncturist Emma Cannon, as well as some of the great doctors in this book. The advice sections at the end of each chapter will give you access to their insights too.

It was such a privilege for me to find out the inner thoughts and lives of the women in the book, to learn how they dealt with sometimes life-and-death issues and came out the other side with more self-knowledge, a little scarred and a little older, but always wiser. It was also often a lot of fun to talk to them and especially good to discover that I could laugh during the dark time after my miscarriage.

Recently, I've read a lot of arguments against IVF, mostly in the context of arguments against the NHS providing it. Some people dismiss couples' and women's wish for a baby, saying that childlessness is a 'social problem', not a medical one and, as such, shouldn't be prioritised. I'm not criticising those who choose not to have children, but isn't it natural that most people do want them? And, if the medical treatment is there, shouldn't people be able to access it?

It's true that IVF is by no means perfect. Most IVF is done at private clinics and there's no limit set on what can be charged, so it's often expensive. And there's also no guarantee of success; if buying a house is the biggest investment most people make, doing IVF is their biggest gamble. But I know I speak for every woman who's been successful due to IVF when I say I'm glad I did it. My gorgeous child wouldn't exist without it, so I will be forever grateful to the scientists who invented it and the doctors who practise it. And I sincerely hope that you'll be able to say the same thing soon.

Further reading

· · · · · · · · · · · ·

Zita West's *Guide to Fertility and Assisted Conception: Essential advice on preparing your body for IVF and other fertility treatments* (Vermilion) answers every question you might have on the nuts and bolts of IVF, including how exactly the drugs work and what to expect from a cycle. *The Complete Guide to IVF: An Inside View of Fertility Clinics and Treatment* by Kate Brian (Piatkus) is another general guide, this time written by a journalist who has experienced IVF herself.

If you like the complementary approach, Emma Cannon's *The Baby-Making Bible: Simple steps to enhance your fertility and improve your chances of getting pregnant* (Rodale) has advice on how to look after yourself properly when you're trying to conceive, from a Chinese medical perspective.

Taking Charge Of Your Fertility: The Definitive Guide to Natural Birth Control, Pregnancy Achievement and Reproductive Health by Toni Weschler (HarperCollins) contains comprehensive instructions by a respected US doctor on how to chart and read your menstrual cycle.

The magazine *Fertility Road* is a good way to keep up to date on new treatments and clinic news (fertilityroad.com).

Websites

The Infertility Network website is a great resource, run by people who really care about helping patients get through fertility treatment (www.infertilitynetworkuk.com).

Fertilityfriends.co.uk, fertilityzone.co.uk and fertility-planit.com are useful resources for finding fertility buddies and personal opinions of clinics.

References

. . . .

1. E. Jedel, F. Labrie, A. Oden, G. Holm, L. Nilsson, P. O., Janson, A.-K. Lind, C. Ohlsson, E. Stener-Victorin, 'Impact of electro-acupuncture and physical exercise on hyperandrogenism and oligo/amenorrhea in women with polycystic ovary syndrome: a randomized controlled trial', *American Journal of Physiology: Endocrinology and Metabolism*, 2010; 300 (1): E37 DOI: 10.1152/ajpendo.00495.2010; http://dx.doi.org/10.1152/ajpendo.00495.2010>
2. Tehrani, F. R., Solaymani-Dodaran, M., Hedayati, M., Azizi, F., 'Is polycystic ovary syndrome an exception for reproductive aging?', *Human Reproduction*, July 2010, 25(7):1775–81; epub 30 April 2010; www.ncbi.nlm.nih.gov/pubmed?term=%22Tehrani%20 FR%22%5BAuthor%5.
3. *Human Reproduction*, DOI: 10.1093/humrep/deq088
4. Showell, M. G., Brown, J., Yazdani, A., Stankiewicz, M. T., Hart. R. J., 'Antioxidants for male subfertility', Cochrane Database of Systematic Reviews 2011, Issue 1, art. no.: CD007411; DOI: 10.1002/14651858.CD007411.pub2.
5. Islam, R., 'Socioeconomic class and smoking linked to premature menopause', European Society of Human Reproduction and Embryology, 6 July 2011.
6. Janvier, A., Spelke, B., Barrington, K., 'The Epidemic of Multiple Gestations and Neonatal Intensive Care Unit Use: The Cost of Irresponsibility', *Journal of Pediatrics*, 14 April 2011; article in press DOI: 10.1016/j.jpeds.2011.02.017
7. Bewley, S., Foo, L., Braude, P., 'Adverse outcomes from IVF', *British Medical Journal*, 2011; 342:d436.

Index

Acknowledgements

• • • • • • • • • • •

F irst thanks must go to all the women in this book, and their husbands and partners, for letting me tell their stories. A huge thank you to my husband Adam for letting me tell our story too.

Thanks to Helena Nicholls, Laura Summers, Helen Hawksfield and everyone at HarperCollins, as well as to Alice Walker, Gill Paul and to my agent Clare Hulton.

Thanks to all the experts who were so generous in providing their time and opinions throughout the book. And to Susan Seenan at IN UK and Nick Spears at the HFEA.

Thanks to my editor at Red, Sam Baker. Big thanks to Helen, Anna, Kate, Camilla, Nikki, Carys, Jo, Lindsay, Saska, Nicola and Amanda for your help, opinions, advice and cheerleading. And a special thank you to my mother, Anna, whose motto 'you can do anything you want to, if you really want to' kept me going.